Common Symptoms in Outpatient Practice

Editor

LIA S. LOGIO

MEDICAL CLINICS OF NORTH AMERICA

www.medical.theclinics.com

Consulting Editor
JACK ENDE

January 2021 • Volume 105 • Number 1

ELSEVIER

1600 John F. Kennedy Boulevard ● Suite 1800 ● Philadelphia, Pennsylvania, 19103-2899

http://www.theclinics.com

MEDICAL CLINICS OF NORTH AMERICA Volume 105, Number 1
January 2021 ISSN 0025-7125, ISBN-13: 978-0-323-79249-3

Editor: Katerina Heidhausen
Developmental Editor: Nick Henderson

Medical Clinics of North America (ISSN 0025-7125) is published bimonthly by Elsevier Inc., 360 Park Avenue South, New York, NY 10010-1710. Months of publication are January, March, May, July, September, and November. Business and editorial offices: 1600 John F. Kennedy Boulevard, Suite 1800, Philadelphia, PA 19103-2899. Periodicals postage paid at New York, NY, and additional mailing offices. Subscription prices are USD $304.00 per year (US individuals), $910.00 per year (US institutions), $100.00 per year (US Students), $381.00 per year (Canadian individuals), $965.00 per year (Canadian institutions), $200.00 per year for (foreign students), $100.00 per year for (Canadian students), $422.00 per year (foreign individuals), and $965.00 per year (foreign institutions). To receive student/resident rate, orders must be accompanied by name of affiliated institution, date of term, and the signature of program/residency coordinator on institution letterhead. Orders will be billed at individual rate until proof of status is received. Foreign air speed delivery is included in all Clinics' subscription prices. All prices are subject to change without notice. **POSTMASTER:** Send address changes to *Medical Clinics of North America*, Elsevier Health Sciences Division, Subscription Customer Service, 3251 Riverport Lane, Maryland Heights, MO 63043. **Customer Service: Telephone: 1-800-654-2452** (U.S. and Canada); **1-314-447-8871** (outside U.S. and Canada). **Fax: 314-447-8029. E-mail: journalscustomerserviceusa@ elsevier.com** (for print support); **journalsonlinesupport-usa@elsevier.com** (for online support).

Reprints. For copies of 100 or more of articles in this publication, please contact the Commercial Reprints Department, Elsevier Inc., 360 Park Avenue South, New York, NY 10010-1710. Tel.: 212-633-3874; Fax: 212-633-3820; E-mail: reprints@elsevier.com.

Medical Clinics of North America is also published in Spanish by McGraw-Hill Interamericana Editores S. A., P.O. Box 5-237, 06500 Mexico, D.F., Mexico.

Medical Clinics of North America is covered in *MEDLINE/PubMed (Index Medicus), Current Contents, ASCA, Excerpta Medica, Science Citation Index,* and *ISI/BIOMED.*

Printed in the United States of America.

PROGRAM OBJECTIVE
The goal of the *Medical Clinics of North America* is to keep practicing physicians up to date with current clinical practice by providing timely articles reviewing the state of the art in patient care.

TARGET AUDIENCE
All practicing physicians and other healthcare professionals.

LEARNING OBJECTIVES
Upon completion of this activity, participants will be able to:
1. Review the concept of deliberate and targeted diagnostic testing to address waste in healthcare.
2. Explain the importance of knowing each patient, how they live, and understanding their value systems and the role it plays in providing care and improving outcomes.
3. Discuss various clinical decision tools and how they aid in the approach to patient care.

ACCREDITATION
The Elsevier Office of Continuing Medical Education (EOCME) is accredited by the Accreditation Council for Continuing Medical Education (ACCME) to provide continuing medical education for physicians.

The EOCME designates this journal-based CME activity for a maximum of 14 *AMA PRA Category 1 Credit*(s)™. Physicians should claim only the credit commensurate with the extent of their participation in the activity.

All other healthcare professionals requesting continuing education credit for this enduring material will be issued a certificate of participation.

DISCLOSURE OF CONFLICTS OF INTEREST
The EOCME assesses conflict of interest with its instructors, faculty, planners, and other individuals who are in a position to control the content of CME activities. All relevant conflicts of interest that are identified are thoroughly vetted by EOCME for fair balance, scientific objectivity, and patient care recommendations. EOCME is committed to providing its learners with CME activities that promote improvements or quality in healthcare and not a specific proprietary business or a commercial interest.

The planning committee, staff, authors and editors listed below have identified no financial relationships or relationships to products or devices they or their spouse/life partner have with commercial interest related to the content of this CME activity:
David Jacob Aizenberg, MD; Brian P. Bosworth, MD; Matthew Chakan, MD, FACP; Regina Chavous-Gibson, MSN, RN; Alia Chisty, MS, MD; Aparna Chopra, MBBS; Joshua A. Davis, MD; Jason C. Dukes, MD, MBA, MS; Jack Ende, MD, MACP; Natalie Farha, MD; Saamia Faruqui, MD; Allison H. Ferris, MD; Kirana Gudi, MD; Katerina Heidhausen; Jennifer Hensley, MD; Stacy Higgins, MD; Marilyn Katz, MD; Sarah Koumtouzoua, MD; Susan Lane, MD; Lia Logio, MD, MACP; Maurice Marcaurd, MD; Megan McGervey, MD; Melissa McNeil, MD, MPH, MACP; Aaron Mills, DO; Catherine Nicastri, MD; Fred N. Pelzman, MD; Liyanage Ashanthi Menaka Perera, MD; Amy L. Shaw, MD; David B. Snell, MD; Meghan Snuckel, MD; Abby Spencer, MD, MS, FACP; Jeyanthi Surendrakumar, Beverly G. Tchang, MD; Judy Tung, MD; Hilary Wagner, DO; Clara Weinstock, DO; Adrienne F. Willard, MD

The planning committee, staff, authors and editors listed below have identified financial relationships or relationships to products or devices they or their spouse/life partner have with commercial interest related to the content of this CME activity:
Leon I. Igel, MD: consultant/advisor for Novo Nordisk A/S

Katherine H. Saunders, MD: consultant/advisor for and she and her spouse/partner own stock and are employed by Intellihealth

UNAPPROVED/OFF-LABEL USE DISCLOSURE
The EOCME requires CME faculty to disclose to the participants;
1. When products or procedures being discussed are off-label, unlabelled, experimental, and/or investigational (not US Food and Drug Administration [FDA] approved); and
2. Any limitations on the information presented, such as data that are preliminary or that represent ongoing research, interim analyses, and/or unsupported opinions. Faculty may discuss information about pharmaceutical agents that is outside of FDA-approved labelling. This information is intended solely for CME and is not intended to promote off-label use of these medications. If you have any questions, contact the medical affairs department of the manufacturer for the most recent prescribing information.

TO ENROLL

To enroll in the *Medical Clinics of North America* Continuing Medical Education program, call customer service at 1-800-654-2452 or sign up online at http://www.theclinics.com/home/cme. The CME program is available to subscribers for an additional annual fee of USD 324.00.

METHOD OF PARTICIPATION

In order to claim credit, participants must complete the following;
1. Complete enrolment as indicated above.
2. Read the activity.
3. Complete the CME Test and Evaluation. Participants must achieve a score of 70% on the test. All CME Tests and Evaluations must be completed online.

CME INQUIRIES/SPECIAL NEEDS

For all CME inquiries or special needs, please contact elsevierCME@elsevier.com.

MEDICAL CLINICS OF NORTH AMERICA

FORTHCOMING ISSUES

March 2021
Rheumatology
Brian Mandell, *Editor*

May 2021
Ophthalmology
Nicholas J. Volpe and Paul Bryar, *Editors*

July 2021
Update in Endocrinology
Silvio Inzucchi, Elizabeth Holt, *Editors*

RECENT ISSUES

November 2020
Cancer Prevention and Screening
Robert A. Smith, Kevin Oeffinger, *Editors*

September 2020
Geriatrics
Danelle Cayea, *Editor*

July 2020
Update in Hospital Medicine
Andrew Dunn, *Editor*

SERIES OF RELATED INTEREST

Primary Care: Clinics in Office Practice
https://www.primarycare.theclinics.com/

Contributors

CONSULTING EDITOR

JACK ENDE, MD, MACP
The Schaeffer Professor of Medicine, Department of Medicine, Perelman School of Medicine of the University of Pennsylvania, Philadelphia, Pennsylvania

EDITOR

LIA S. LOGIO, MD, MACP
Professor of Medicine, Case Western Reserve University School of Medicine, Cleveland, Ohio

AUTHORS

DAVID JACOB AIZENBERG, MD
Associate Professor of Clinical Medicine, Department of Medicine, Perelman School of Medicine at the University of Pennsylvania, Philadelphia, Pennsylvania

BRIAN P. BOSWORTH, MD, FACG
Chief of Medicine, NYU Langone Health Main Campus, Tisch Hospital, Professor of Medicine, NYU Grossman School of Medicine New York, New York

MATTHEW CHAKAN, MD, FACP
Assistant Professor, Internal Medicine Department, Eastern Virginia Medical School, Norfolk, Virginia

ALIA CHISTY, MS, MD
Associate Professor of Medicine, Division of General Internal Medicine, Penn State College of Medicine, Penn State Health Milton S. Hershey Medical Center, Hershey, Pennsylvania

APARNA CHOPRA, MBBS
Fellow, Institute for Critical Care Medicine, The Mount Sinai Hospital, New York, New York

JOSHUA A. DAVIS, MD
Pulmonary and Critical Care Fellow, Division of Pulmonary and Critical Care Medicine, New York-Presbyterian Hospital, Weill Cornell Campus, New York, New York

JASON C. DUKES, MD, MBA, MSc
Assistant Professor, Internal Medicine Department, Eastern Virginia Medical School, Norfolk, Virginia

NATALIE FARHA, MD
Internal Medicine, Resident, Cleveland Clinic, Cleveland, Ohio

SAAMIA FARUQUI, MD
Fellow, Division of Gastroenterology and Hepatology, Department of Medicine, New York University, New York, New York

ALLISON H. FERRIS, MD, FACP
Associate Professor of Medicine, Program Director, Internal Medicine Residency, Charles E. Schmidt College of Medicine, Florida Atlantic University, Boca Raton, Florida

KIRANA GUDI, MD
Assistant Professor of Medicine, Weill Department of Medicine, Weill Cornell Medicine, New York, New York

JENNIFER HENSLEY, MD
Assistant Professor, Department of Medicine, Renaissance School of Medicine at SUNY Stony Brook, Stony Brook University Hospital, Stony Brook, New York

STACY HIGGINS, MD, FACP
Professor of Medicine, Division of General Medicine and Geriatrics, Emory University School of Medicine, Atlanta, Georgia

LEON I. IGEL, MD, FACP, FTOS
Assistant Professor, Department of Internal Medicine, Division of Endocrinology, Weill Cornell Medical College, New York, New York

MARILYN KATZ, MD
Associate Professor, Department of Medicine, University of Connecticut School of Medicine, Farmington, Connecticut

SARAH KOUMTOUZOUA, MD
Assistant Professor of Medicine, Division of General Medicine and Geriatrics, Emory University School of Medicine, Atlanta, Georgia

SUSAN LANE, MD
Professor, Department of Medicine, Renaissance School of Medicine at SUNY Stony Brook, Stony Brook University Hospital, Stony Brook, New York

MAURICE MARCAURD, MD
Chief Medical Resident, Internal Medicine Department, Eastern Virginia Medical School, Norfolk, Virginia

MEGAN McGERVEY, MD
Director of Clinical Reasoning and Career Development, Internal Medicine Residency Program, Department of Internal Medicine, Cleveland Clinic, Cleveland, Ohio

MELISSA McNEIL, MD, MPH, MACP
Professor of Medicine and Obstetrics, Gynecology and Reproductive Sciences, University of Pittsburgh, Pittsburgh, Pennsylvania

AARON MILLS, DO
Assistant Professor, Internal Medicine Department, Eastern Virginia Medical School, Norfolk, Virginia

CATHERINE NICASTRI, MD
Associate Professor, Department of Medicine, Renaissance School of Medicine at SUNY Stony Brook, Stony Brook University Hospital, Stony Brook, New York

FRED N. PELZMAN, MD
Associate Professor of Clinical Medicine, Division of General Internal Medicine, Department of Medicine, Weill Cornell Medicine, New York, New York

LIYANAGE ASHANTHI MENAKA PERERA, MD
Senior Associate Consultant, Department of Medicine, Division of Hospital Internal Medicine, Mayo Clinic, Austin, Minnesota

KATHERINE H. SAUNDERS, MD
Assistant Professor, Department of Internal Medicine, Division of Endocrinology, Weill Cornell Medical College, New York, New York

AMY L. SHAW, MD
Assistant Professor of Clinical Medicine, Department of Medicine, Division of Geriatrics and Palliative Medicine, Weill Cornell Medicine, New York, New York

DAVID B. SNELL, MD
Fellow, Division of Gastroenterology and Hepatology, Department of Medicine, New York University, New York, New York

MEGHAN SNUCKEL, MD
Department of Medicine, University of Connecticut School of Medicine, Farmington, Connecticut

ABBY SPENCER, MD, MS, FACP
Program Director, Internal Medicine Residency Program, Associate Professor of Medicine, CCLCM of Case Western Reserve University, Cleveland Clinic, Cleveland, Ohio

BEVERLY G. TCHANG, MD
Assistant Professor, Department of Internal Medicine, Division of Endocrinology, Weill Cornell Medical College, New York, New York

JUDY TUNG, MD
Associate Professor of Clinical Medicine, Division of General Internal Medicine, Department of Medicine, Weill Cornell Medicine, New York, New York

HILARY WAGNER, DO
Department of Medicine, University of Connecticut School of Medicine, Farmington, Connecticut

CLARA WEINSTOCK, DO
Assistant Professor, Department of Medicine, University of Connecticut School of Medicine, Farmington, Connecticut

ADRIENNE F. WILLARD, MD
Associate Professor of Medicine, Drexel University College of Medicine, Philadelphia, Pennsylvania

Contents

Insomnia is a common condition affecting approximately 50% of people at some point. Physicians must be equipped to diagnose and treat it as part of outpatient practice. Chronic insomnia is a common complaint that has potentially dangerous short-term and long-term effects, but effective treatments are available. The 2 methods of treatment are psychological, which is preferred, and pharmacologic, for when behavioral therapies are not effective. It is important to understand the various behavioral interventions and risks and benefits of the medications available to engage patients in a shared decision-making model to find the best treatment for each patient.

Knee pain is present in up to 20% of the adult general population and can be significantly debilitating to patients. A thorough history and physical examination can help localize the source of inflammation or injury to further determine if imaging, physical therapy, specialty referral, or surgery is necessary. By following a systematic approach to evaluating knee pain, primary care physicians can make the correct diagnosis and formulate an appropriate therapeutic strategy for patients.

Owing to the broad differential diagnoses that can present as fatigue, a rational approach to diagnosis is paramount. Performance of a battery of diagnostic tests is unlikely to assist with diagnosis, highlighting the importance of a thorough history and physical examination. Fatigue can be a sequela of an underlying medical disease or exists as a primary condition. Management of secondary fatigue largely depends on treatment of the underlying condition. There are no FDA-approved medications for primary fatigue, now known as system exertion intolerance disease. Treatment is focused on individualized exercise therapy and cognitive behavioral therapy.

Obesity is a chronic disease caused by dysregulated energy homeostasis pathways that encourage the accumulation of adiposity, which in turn results in the development or exacerbation of weight-related comorbidities. Treatment of obesity relies on a foundation of lifestyle modification; weight loss pharmacotherapy, bariatric surgery and devices are additional tools to help patients achieve their health goals. Appropriate management of patients with obesity provides multiple metabolic benefits beyond weight loss.

Foreword
Nine "C's" and Counting

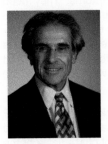

Jack Ende, MD, MACP
Consulting Editor

The late and legendary Barbara Starfield captured the essence of primary care with her alliterative chestnut: The Four C's. Primary care, she asserted, should provide patients with care that is: first Contact, Comprehensive, Continuous, and Coordinated. She developed this model in 1992, almost 30 years ago. Since then, others have expanded upon the Four C's, for example, Doerr and colleagues[1] took us up to 9 C's, adding Credible, meaning the primary care provider earns the patient's trust; Collaborative, acknowledging that good primary care often depends on integrated systems; Cost-effective, which can be considered synonymous with High-Value Care; Capacity expansion, indicating that effective primary care amplifies the physician workforce by referring to specialists only when necessary; and Career satisfaction, which I note is a theme appropriately echoed by Dr Logio, our Guest Editor, when she notes that, "intentionally elegant diagnostic care" can be an antidote to burnout. I agree. I am happiest when I fully understand the problems my patients bring to me and am confident that even if I cannot relieve their symptoms, I am going about the workup in the proper way and have a well-tested approach for their problem. I don't feel confused; I feel in control. I have a sense of competency.

Competency, I believe, is the difference between, on the one hand, frustration and doubt and, on the other hand, satisfaction and certainty. It is the difference between burnout and joy. At the risk of sounding biblical, and with all deference to the Old Testament, I propose Competence as the tenth C.

How is Competence manifested in primary care? Not necessarily by encyclopedic, highly detailed knowledge, nor by exhaustive differential diagnoses for the common problems our patients bring to us. No. Competence in symptom management depends more on having a method, that is, an approach. And so, it is interesting to see how many of the 14 articles in this issue, *Common Symptoms in Outpatient Practice*, use *approach* in the title. "An Approach to the Patient with Cough;" "Current Approach to Constipation;" and an approach to knee pain, fatigue, weight

Med Clin N Am 105 (2021) xv–xvi
https://doi.org/10.1016/j.mcna.2020.10.008
0025-7125/21/© 2020 Published by Elsevier Inc.

loss, and so forth. Having an approach is the difference between ordering a slew of tests for, say, anemia, versus sorting things out at the very outset with an algorithm that distinguishes blood loss from decreased production, or evaluating hyponatremia based upon volume status. That is what primary care physicians need to bring to their encounters, and that is what the authors assembled by Dr Logio provide.

Primary care physicians need approaches to common symptoms. They need methods, not minutia. Perhaps Osler said it best in his advice regarding clinical education: "The problem with medical students is that they try to learn too much; the problem with medical educators is that they try to teach too much. Teach them methods and the art of observation, and then give them patients to practice their skills." That is what we should be providing for our students, and that is what we should be focusing on for ourselves.

Jack Ende, MD, MACP
Department of Medicine
Perelman School of Medicine of the
University of Pennsylvania
5033 W. Gates Pavilion
3400 Spruce Street
Philadelphia, PA 19104, USA

E-mail address:
jack.ende@pennmedicine.upenn.edu

REFERENCES

1. Doerr, et al. The Accountable Primary Care Model: Beyond Medical Home 2.0. AMAC 2014;2(4):54–62.

Preface

Common Symptoms in Outpatient Practice

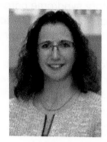

Lia S. Logio, MD, MACP
Editor

Welcome to this issue of *Medical Clinics of North America* focused on Common Symptoms in Outpatient Practice. We hope you find this a valuable resource to the most common complaints seen in your practice.

We focused on the best up-to-date evidence on prevalence, test characteristics, and elegant diagnostic processes. Our patients deserve the best quality for the lowest cost and harm (ie, high-value care). We sought to provide very practical advice about eliminating unnecessary tests and health care waste.

You will notice a few very important themes across these articles. The first is the focus on the patient. It is clear that best practice in approaching patients is to know them. Know the way they live, what they value, how they spend their time, what they fear. It is in building a strong relationship with each individual that you will provide the best care, navigating with them what the underlying cause is and the best strategy for improving their symptoms and helping them live a fully healthy life. It cannot be overemphasized and reminds us of Francis Peabody's famous quote, *"One of the essential qualities of the clinician is interest in humanity, for the secret of the care of the patient is in caring for the patient."*

Second, we were very deliberate in recommending testing only where it will add value to the patient's experience. We are all responsible for addressing the waste in health care, including duplicate testing and overtesting. It is better for the patients and for the system to be targeted and to use your expertise to narrow down possibilities.

Third, we sought to include important clinical tools that will help you in your approach to the patient. There are tables, clinical decision tools, and even a few videos included in this issue.

I will close by reaffirming my belief that the relationship-centered intentionally elegant diagnostic approach to doctoring is the antidote to three ailments in health

Med Clin N Am 105 (2021) xvii–xviii
https://doi.org/10.1016/j.mcna.2020.10.007
0025-7125/21/© 2020 Published by Elsevier Inc.

care: the burnout epidemic in health care providers, the paucity of new physicians choosing to practice primary care, and the fragmentation of our system, which remains challenged to provide the best coordinated and comprehensive care our patients deserve.

The authors of the enclosed articles are all medical educators who regularly give of their time and talent to educate patients, communities, and learners at every level. I am proud to call them friends and colleagues. Even more impressive is the fact that this issue was produced during the peak of the severe acute respiratory syndrome coronavirus2 global pandemic when many of these individuals were front-line caregivers to sick patients and overloaded systems. I'm in awe of their commitment and perseverance in the face of long days with an uncertain end.

Ultimately, caring is a form of love. As physicians, we care for so many: our families, our learners, our communities, our patients. We must also care for ourselves and strive to always find ways of bringing joy and meaning into our simple daily tasks. Inspire others to do the same.

Happy reading!

Lia S. Logio, MD, MACP
Professor of Medicine
Case Western Reserve University
School of Medicine
Cleveland, OH, USA

E-mail addresses:
drlialogio@gmail.com; lxl789@case.edu

Evaluating and Managing the Patient with Back Pain

Sarah Koumtouzoua, MD, Stacy Higgins, MD*

KEYWORDS

- Outpatient • Nontraumatic • Red flags • Diagnostics • Therapy • Prognosis

KEY POINTS

- The history and physical examination should be used to direct any diagnostic testing in the evaluation of low back pain (LBP) in adults.
- The presence of red flags on history or physical examination should trigger early ordering of imaging studies.
- Use of a diagnostic algorithm can direct which imaging tests should be part of the initial evaluation.
- Most acute back pain will resolve without therapeutic intervention.
- In care of the patient with LBP, adherence to high-value principles and evidenced-based practice will help control cost and lead to improved outcomes.

LOW BACK PAIN
Case Study

A 62-year-old woman with history of chronic kidney disease, hypertension, and depression presents with 2 weeks of acute worsening of her chronic low back pain (LBP). Previous radiographic imaging showed degenerative joint disease with joint space narrowing in the L4-L5 region. She denies leg weakness or falls but does have occasional radiation of sharp pain down her right posterior leg, without associated saddle anesthesia or incontinence of urine or feces. She denies recent trauma or injuries and notes that the pain is worse with walking and improved with sitting and leaning forward while walking. She has tried acetaminophen and a lumbar back support with minimal relief.

Review of systems is negative for weight loss, night sweats, fevers, or fatigue. Medications are amlodipine and losartan. She works in a warehouse, but had difficulty completing her tasks and requested light duty in order to avoid increased activity and pain. She does not use tobacco, alcohol, or illicit drugs.

Division of General Medicine and Geriatrics, Emory University School of Medicine, 49 Jesse Hill Jr. Drive Southeast, Suite 407, Atlanta, GA 30303, USA
* Corresponding author.
E-mail address: smhiggi@emory.edu

Med Clin N Am 105 (2021) 1–17
https://doi.org/10.1016/j.mcna.2020.08.014
0025-7125/21/© 2020 Elsevier Inc. All rights reserved.

Examination is remarkable for a positive straight-leg raise on the right, 5/5 strength in the bilateral upper and lower extremities with intact sensation to light touch throughout, 2+ patellar and Achilles reflexes on the right, 3+ on the left, with down-going Babinski bilaterally.

Although she has had this pain for several years, she has never completed physical therapy or undergone any invasive interventions. She is frustrated and states that her pain and disability affect her mood. She would like to "know what's causing this" and "fix it" so that she can return to working without restrictions.

Background/Epidemiology

Back pain is one of the most common complaints seen in the United States. In estimates from 2 national surveys conducted by the National Center for Health Statistics in 2002, back pain was the most frequent type of pain reported by civilian, noninstitutionalized adult respondents. More than 25% of respondents reported having LBP within the prior 3 months, corresponding to an estimated 54 million adults, and a reported lifetime prevalence of nearly 80%. LBP accounted for approximately 2.3% of all office visits, and it is the fifth most common reason for all physician visits in the United States.[1]

Back pain has imposed significant costs on the US health care system. Using data from the 1998 Medical Expenditure Panel Survey, it was found that health care expenditures on back pain were approximately $91 billion, with $28 billion for inpatient care and $23.6 billion for office-based visits. Other costs included prescription drugs, outpatient service, emergency department visits, and home health services. These expenditures do not include indirect costs from lost work, which are estimated to be substantial. Individuals with back pain were found to incur total health expenditures about 1.6-fold more than individuals without back pain. Among patients with a primary diagnosis of LBP, 10% of individuals accounted for close to 100% of the inpatient expenditures, 90% of emergency department visits, and 87% of outpatient services.[2]

This review focuses on the target population of adults with LBP that is nontraumatic in nature.

Definitions

In evaluation and treatment of LBP, categorizing and identifying the chronicity is most important in guiding decision making, including the appropriate diagnostic workup and the most effective management. LBP can be sorted into 3 categories: acute, LBP being present for less than 4 weeks; subacute, present for anywhere from 4 weeks to 3 months; or chronic/persistent LBP.[3] Recurrent back pain has variable definitions in the literature, taking into account number of episodes, frequency, duration, and severity. Most commonly included is frequency of previous episodes, although that might range anywhere from pain at least once a year to pain twice over a lifetime.[4] As such, in discussing management of recurrent LBP, it should be treated as chronic.

History and Physical Examination

There are 2 key questions that the history and physical examination can help assess: (a) Is there a serious systemic disease causing the pain? and (b) Is there neurologic compromise that might require surgical evaluation? A focused and well-performed history and physical examination can help triage whether further imaging and diagnostics are needed. The presence of any of the red flags listed in **Table 1** on history or physical examination would indicate the need for further diagnostic evaluation.

Initial history questions should include pain location, associated symptoms, character of the pain, alleviating (including over-the-counter medications) and aggravating

Table 1	
RED FLAGS requiring further diagnostics	
History Red Flags	**Physical Examination Red Flags**
• History of cancer (+LR 14.7 for cancer)	• Fever
• Corticosteroid use	• Motor weakness in legs
• History of osteoporosis	• Sensory level or
• Abnormal neurologic history,	saddle anesthesia
new falls, ataxia, >3 wk of midline pain,	• Diminished or
nocturnal pain, sphincter incontinence or	abnormal reflexes,
urinary urgency, bilateral leg symptoms	including positive Babinski
• Anticoagulant use	• Fecal incontinence
• Intravenous drug use	• Urinary retention
• Fever	
• Immunocompromised	
• Unexplained weight loss (+LR 2.7)	
• Recent spinal anesthesia	
• Failure to improve after 1 mo (+LR 3.0)	
• Age >70	

factors, timing and duration of symptoms, pain severity, history of similar symptoms, and past treatments used. It is also important to consider psychosocial factors (so-called yellow flags): presence of depression, passive coping strategies, job dissatisfaction, higher disability levels, disputed compensation claims, and somatization. The focused physical examination should begin with inspection of the back with attention to the area of discomfort, followed by direct palpation of the spine and paraspinal muscles. Assessment of range of motion (flexion/extension, rotation, lateral bend) and gait is helpful for impact on daily activities. These factors may have an impact on likelihood and time to recovery.

Risk factors for potential serious conditions that would require further diagnostic evaluation are outlined in **Table 1** and should be assessed in all patients. Historically, isolated age greater than 50 without other risk factors has been identified as a red flag requiring further diagnostics despite the lack of evidence supporting this recommendation. In 2015, a prospective study of 5239 patients with LBP older than the age of 65 was conducted, evaluating differences in outcomes at 1 year. They found no difference in reports of disability, but marked differences in cost and resource use. In addition, there were no significant differences seen in missed diagnoses, such as malignancy or infection.[5]

Differential Diagnoses

Most LBP is due to nonspecific musculoskeletal strain, and episodes generally resolve within days to a few weeks with self-care. Up to one-third of patients report persistent back pain of at least moderate intensity 1 year after an acute episode.[6] In considering the differential for LBP, a focused history and physical examination will help to categorize patients into one of the groupings listed in **Table 2**.

More than 90% of symptomatic lumbar disc herniations occur at the L4/L5 and L5/S1 levels. History that supports disc herniation includes worsened pain with maneuvers that increase intraabdominal pressure, including coughing, sneezing, or straining, along with pain and numbness in the corresponding nerve distribution. On physical examination, assessment of L4-L5 and L5-S1 motor strength is assessed by squatting and rising (L4) and walking on heels (L5) and toes (S1). Loss of patellar (L4) and Achilles

Table 2	
Differential diagnosis, low back pain	
• Nonspecific LBP	1. Degenerative spine disease 2. Muscular or ligamentous injury
• Back pain with radiculopathy or spinal stenosis	1. Acute disc herniation 2. Spinal stenosis
• Other spinal pathologic condition	1. Metastatic epidural tumor 2. Spinal epidural abscess 3. Osteomyelitis 4. Infectious discitis 5. Epidural hematoma 6. Central disc herniation with cauda equina syndrome 7. Compression fracture 8. Ankylosing spondylitis
• Extraspinal pathologic conditions	1. Aortic aneurysm 2. Cholangitis 3. Shingles 4. Pneumonia 5. Pancreatitis 6. Nephrolithiasis

(S1) reflexes also points toward disc herniation. The straight-leg raise test can assess for nerve-root compression at these levels. It is described as positive when passive elevation of the leg by cupping the heel reproduces pain radiating down the posterior leg below the knee at between 30° and 70°. A positive ipsilateral straight-leg-raise test has a sensitivity of 64% and specificity of 57%, whereas a crossed straight-leg-raise test has a sensitivity of 28% and specificity of 90%.[7]

Spinal stenosis is a common source of LBP and impaired walking in patients older than 65 years old. The most common cause is related to age-associated degeneration of the lumbar disks and facet joints, leading to disk height loss and associated disk bulging. Patients present with symptoms of pseudo-claudication or neurogenic claudication, defined as leg pain that radiates into the buttocks and/or the thigh and lower leg, worsened with prolonged walking and improved with sitting. Pain is exacerbated by lumbar extension and improved with lumbar flexion.[8]

The most common manifestation of osteoporosis is vertebral fractures, seen with increasing prevalence and incidence with advanced age, and in white women over black women, Asian women, or men. Most vertebral fractures are incidentally identified on radiographs without accompanying clinical symptoms. In premenopausal women who present with incident vertebral fracture, it is important to assess for other clinical risk factors, such as prior fracture, fall, inactivity, tobacco use, systemic glucocorticoid use, low body mass index, or medical history of chronic obstructive pulmonary disease, seropositive rheumatoid arthritis, and Crohn disease.[9]

Infections of the spine include epidural abscess, discitis, and osteomyelitis. Infections are usually blood-borne, a result of direct inoculation at the time of spinal surgery, or contiguous spread from adjacent soft tissue that is infected.[10] The authors have seen increasing incidence of spinal infections over the last 30 years with an aging population, higher numbers of immunocompromised hosts and intravenous drug users, and increased spinal procedures. In the primary care setting, outside of localized back pain, the presenting signs and symptoms of spinal infection are nonspecific and limited to fever and decreased range of motion.[11]

Imaging and Additional Testing

Further diagnostic workup of LBP is often not indicated, nor supported by evidence because acute to subacute nonspecific LBP will resolve spontaneously in two-thirds of cases.[12] High-value care supports the use of historical and physical examination findings to guide treatment and management of LBP, with low yield in pursuing further diagnostic workup in the absence of clinical red flags or suspicion of serious pathologic condition in the first 4 to 6 weeks of symptoms.[13] Routine imaging without evidence of progressive neurologic deficits or signs and symptoms of a serious or specific underlying condition, such as malignancy, inflammation, or infection, does not contribute clinically beneficial information and can lead to unnecessary harm.[14] In considering whether and which type of imaging may be indicated in the acute setting, the authors recommend use of the Appropriateness Criteria, an imaging guideline compiled by the American College of Radiology in coordination with other society experts, which provides recommendations that balance imaging utility, harms, and costs.[12]

Radiography has a high rate of false positives in testing and overall is more difficult to interpret. Degenerative changes are often evident on plain film, particularly with advancing age, but these findings are not clinically significant in most situations because they are reported equally in both symptomatic and asymptomatic persons.[15] As detailed in **Fig. 1**, radiography is recommended in the initial evaluation if the patient has a history of low-velocity trauma, osteoporosis, or chronic steroid use along with workup of LBP in younger patients with suspicion for spondylolysis or inflammatory arthritis.[12] Radiography should not be used for evaluation of red flags given its poor sensitivity.[12]

Computed tomography (CT) is not as sensitive for soft tissue concerns, such as discitis or myelopathy, but is more useful in the diagnosis of fractures, dislocations, spondylolisthesis, scoliosis, stenosis, and tumors.[15] In patients who have contraindications to MRI imaging, CT with myelography is an alternative for spinal canal imaging in cases of myelopathies with progressively worsening neurologic function or concern for cauda equine syndrome (CES).[12] For patients who meet high-risk criteria for cervical vertebral injury as defined by the Canadian Cervical Rules, particularly in the posterior column where x-ray has low sensitivity, CT without contrast is the preferred imaging modality in order to properly evaluate fractures.[12] No validated tools exist to guide decision making for further imaging of suspected thoracolumbar spinal injuries; therefore, there should be a low threshold to obtain imaging, given the low sensitivity of physical examination to detect spinal injuries[16] (**Table 3**).

MRI is the most sensitive and specific imaging modality of choice for diagnosing neurologic conditions causing LBP because of the ability to delineate the relationship of disc to nerve, along with the visualization of soft tissue and bony structures. Because of its high sensitivity, MRI often detects asymptomatic disc herniations and protrusions.[15] MRI remains the recommended imaging of choice per the Appropriateness Criteria in the workup for red flags and in the evaluation of persistent or progressive symptoms following 6 weeks of conservative therapy whereby there remains diagnostic uncertainty. MRI is also recommended to evaluate the anatomy for potential invasive interventions to treat radicular pain.[12] Depending on the red flag, contrast may or may not be needed, as detailed in **Fig. 1**. It is more sensitive and specific than CT in detecting spinal pathologic conditions, such as inflammation, infection, and tumors, allowing for earlier detection of osteomyelitis, discitis, epidural infections, and hematomas. MRI with contrast can detect both malignant bone lesions and infection before bone erosion is detectable on either CT or radiography.[12] In cases of suspected

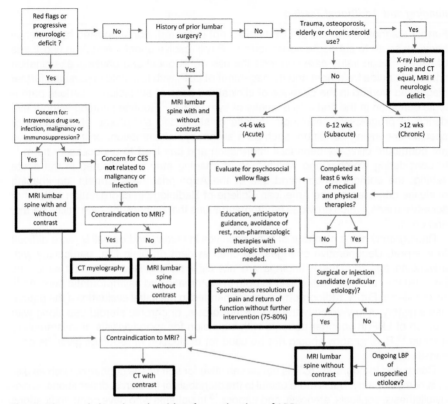

Fig. 1. Diagnostic imaging algorithm for evaluation of LBP.

Table 3	
Canadian cervical rules for suspected cervical spine injury	
High-Risk Factors	**Low-Risk Factors**
Presence of 1 high-risk criterion indicates need for automatic imaging of cervical spine and immobilization of the cervical spine until completed	Presence of 1 or more low-risk factors allows for deferment of screening imaging. Completion of examination with rotation of head 45° past midline in both directions clears patient of cervical spinal injury and need for imaging

• Age>65 y
• Paresthesias in extremities
• Dangerous mechanism:
  ○ Fall from >3 ft/5 stairs
  ○ Axial load to head
  ○ Motor vehicle crash with high speed, rollover, or ejection
  ○ Bicycle collision
  ○ Motorized recreational vehicle accident
	• Simple rear-end motor vehicle crash
	• Patient in sitting position on examination
	• Patient ambulatory any time after trauma
	• Delayed onset of pain
	• Absence of midline cervical spine tenderness

CES or progressive neurologic decline, it is more appropriate to use MRI without contrast rather than with contrast.[12]

There is no utility of imaging studies in the workup of uncomplicated, nonspecific, chronic LBP unless there remains diagnostic uncertainty. Repeat imaging is also not likely to detect changes in disc disease and should not be done unless there is a concerning new red flag or neurologic change on physical examination.[12]

Serum Studies/Other Workup

Laboratory assessment should be guided by history and physical examination findings that raise diagnostic concern for systemic pathologic conditions as the cause of LBP, both intraspinal and extraspinal. Serum studies, such as erythrocyte sedimentation rate, C-reactive protein, and complete blood count, can aid in evaluating for inflammatory or infectious processes. Studies, such as urinalysis, liver function tests, and lipase, can be helpful for assessing extraspinal sources of back pain. Evaluating calcium and alkaline phosphatase levels may be useful in the diagnosis of spinal malignancies.[17]

Evidence-Based Therapeutic Options

Regardless of acuity and duration, nonpharmacologic approaches should be prioritized over pharmacologic and invasive treatment modalities,[18] but particularly in the case of chronic pain.[13] Most clinical guidelines agree that nonpharmacologic interventions, such as maintaining activity, education/reassurance, exercise therapy, and cognitive behavioral therapy, should be first-line treatments, over pharmacologic and invasive therapies, such as spinal injections, radiofrequency denervation, or surgery.[19] In systematic reviews and guidelines on treatment of LBP that have examined outcomes on pain and function related to interventions, no one individual modality shows large, long-term effects to decrease pain or improve function and reduce disability with any of the commonly recommended pharmacologic and nonpharmacologic therapies used for management.[18]

Nonpharmacologic interventions

Acute back pain Most episodes of acute back pain will resolve spontaneously within 1 month, with most patients not seeking medical care. For those who present for care, guidelines agree that acute, nonspecific LBP should first be treated with reassurance of a favorable prognosis. Recommendations should focus on minimal interventions and resumption of normal activities, with the avoidance of bed rest.[13]

Nonpharmacologic interventions, such as superficial heat and massage, acupuncture, or spinal manipulation, should be used first if choosing a treatment. Comparisons of efficacy of pain reduction, functional improvement, and strength of evidence of various nonpharmacologic interventions are listed in **Table 4**.[18]

Chronic back pain As with acute LBP, nonpharmacologic treatment options should be offered first in chronic back pain, along with recommendations to avoid bedrest and limits to normal activities.[13] Nonpharmacologic treatments that should be offered include exercise, multidisciplinary rehabilitation, acupuncture, mindfulness-based stress reduction, tai chi, yoga, motor control exercise, progressive relaxation, electromyography (EMG) biofeedback, cognitive-based therapy (CBT), or spinal manipulation.[18] Therapies with no benefit in pain reduction or improvement in function with chronic LBP include massage, ultrasound, transcutaneous electrical nerve stimulation (TENS), lumbar support, or taping.[18]

Most guidelines recommend the use of psychological therapies, particularly in the case of chronic LBP and in cases where psychosocial "yellow flags" are identified.[13]

Table 4
Comparisons of nonpharmacologic treatments and their use in acute-subacute low back pain with reduction in pain, disability, and associated harm as rated by quality of evidence

Therapy Type	Magnitude of Pain Reduction	Magnitude of Functional Improvement	Harm Associated with Treatment	Strength of Evidence	Notes
Superficial heat therapy	**	**	Increased skin flushing	**	Exceeds NSAIDs, acetaminophen for pain
Acupuncture	*	—	None	*	Exceeds NSAIDs for pain
Massage	**	**	Soreness during or after	*	Short-term (1 wk) effects
Chiropractic spinal manipulation	—	*	Muscle soreness, increase in pain	*	Short-term (1 wk) effects
Lumbar support	—	—	None	*	
Exercise therapy	—	—	Muscle soreness, increased pain	*	

Ordered from highest quality evidence, most difference to lowest.
***,high; **, moderate; *, small; —, no effect.

Comparison of evidence supporting the efficacy of various nonpharmacologic interventions in the treatment of chronic LBP is listed in **Table 5**.[20]

Pharmacologic interventions
Acute back pain In the acute phase of LBP if pharmacologic treatments are desired, the lowest effective dose of short-course nonsteroidal anti-inflammatory drugs (NSAIDs) or skeletal muscle relaxants (SMRs) should be chosen as first-line therapy.[18] Acetaminophen has been previously recommended as first-line pharmacologic treatment of LBP, but recent evidence shows no benefit over placebo or when compared with NSAIDs.[18] Other therapies, such as antidepressants, benzodiazepines, anticonvulsants, and opioids, have insufficient evidence to support their use[18] (**Table 6**).

Chronic back pain In evaluating treatments for chronic back pain, pharmacologic options for treatment provide moderate at best, and often only small improvements in pain for short amounts of time, with minimal effects on function and disability. In addition, it is unclear if pain reduction using these medications provides a clinically significant difference in outcome. Furthermore, the combination of therapies or sequence of their use has not been well studied.[21] Studies on pharmacologic treatment of radicular back pain have not had sufficient evidence to suggest 1 therapy over another, including evaluation of NSAIDs, anticonvulsants, and serotonin and norepinehprine reuptake inhibitors (SNRIs).

In chronic LBP, only those with an inadequate response to nonpharmacologic interventions should pursue pharmacologic treatment, with NSAIDs as first-line therapy and duloxetine or tramadol as second-line therapy.[21]

Opioids should only be used after a risk-benefit discussion with the patient and if all other treatments have failed.[18] There are no long-term evaluations on effectiveness and harm for the use of opioids in the treatment of chronic LBP.[21]

Other therapies found to be ineffective or insufficient evidence to support their use include tricyclic antidepressants, selective serotonin reuptake inhibitors (SSRIs), SMRs, systemic corticosteroids, or anticonvulsant medications.

Very little evidence exists to support specific treatments for radicular or intrinsic spinal-related LBP, including recommendations for systemic pharmacologic treatments. The only reliable recommendation based on evidence for improvement in pain related to radicular back pain is exercise therapy.[18]

Topical analgesics
Topical analgesics for the management of LBP are lacking evidence, but may be of use with acute lumbar musculoskeletal strains. Topical NSAIDs when rubbed on skin can reduce pain by 50% in about a week in approximately 20% to 50% of patients with acute musculoskeletal strain. There is no evidence to support the use of other types of topical analgesics for other causes or durations of LBP.[22]

Invasive/interventional
Most guidelines recommend against invasive measures, such as epidural steroid injections and surgery, for treatment of nonspecific LBP. There is limited comparison evidence looking at the use of nonpharmacologic interventions versus invasive and interventional methods.[21]

Epidural corticosteroid injections could be considered in cases of chronic radiculopathies and radicular pain that has not responded to conservative measures, as there is evidence supporting that they create immediate and short-term (<3 months) reductions in pain and improvement in function. Injections did not create a long-term reduction in risk for surgery, and they have not been shown to benefit patients with spinal

Table 5
Comparisons of nonpharmacologic treatments and their use in chronic low back pain with reduction in pain, disability, and associated harm as rated by quality of evidence

Therapy Type	Magnitude of Pain Reduction	Magnitude of Functional Improvement	Harm Associated with Treatment	Strength of Evidence	Notes
Multidisciplinary rehabilitation	**	*	None	**	Long-term effects on pain small
Acupuncture	**	**	None	**	Greater effect on pain, function than NSAIDs
Mindfulness-based stress reduction^	*	*	None	**	Easy to access, low cost
Exercise therapies	*	*	Muscle soreness, increased pain, injury	**	All exercise therapies are equal
Progressive relaxation^	**	**	None	*	Equal to CBT, mindfulness-based stress reduction
Yoga	**	**	Mild muscle soreness	*	Greater effects on pain than exercise
Tai chi	**	*	None	*	Greater effects on pain than exercise
Motor control exercise	**	*	None	*	Greater effects on pain, function than exercise or physical therapy
CBT^	**	—	None	*	Equal to mindfulness-based stress reduction
EMG biofeedback^	**	—	None	*	Equal to other psychological therapies
Spinal manipulation	*	—	Muscle soreness and increased pain, injury	*	

***, high; **, moderate; *, small; —, no effect; ^, psychological therapy.
Ordered from highest-quality evidence, most difference to lowest.

Table 6
Comparisons of systemic pharmacologic treatments and their use in acute low back pain with reduction in pain, disability, and associated harm as rated by quality of evidence

Therapy Type	Magnitude of Pain Reduction	Magnitude of Functional Improvement	Harm Associated with Treatment	Quality of Evidence
NSAIDs	*	*	More adverse events	**
SMRs	*	—	Increased sedation, central nervous system events	**
Systemic corticosteroids	—	—	Increased risk of insomnia, nervousness, increased appetite	*
Acetaminophen	—	—	No adverse events	*
Benzodiazepines	Unable to estimate	Unable to estimate	More frequent somnolence, fatigue, lightheadedness	Insufficient
Antiepileptics-gabapentin/pregabalin	No evidence	No evidence	No clear adverse events	
Opioids	No evidence	No evidence	Increased nausea, dizziness, constipation, vomiting, somnolence, dry mouth, dependence	

***,high; **, moderate; *, small; —, no effect.

stenosis.[23] Evaluation of injections as part of a broader pain management strategy has not been well studied, along with approaches, doses, and use in varying severities of radicular pain.[23] Similar to epidural injection, radiofrequency denervation has only small and short-term effects on pain and function. Facet joint injections and trigger point injections have no benefit.[24]

Discectomy should only be considered for severe chronic LBP owing to disk herniation that has failed conservative management. Spinal fusion surgeries should also be deferred to carefully selected cases of severe LBP that have failed 2 years of active rehabilitation programs. Surgical intervention for spinal stenosis has no benefits and should be avoided with the exception of severe stenosis with progressive neurologic deficits and neurogenic claudication.[24]

Risks for Development of Chronic Back Pain/Prognosis

In managing both acute and chronic LBP, guidelines recommend that clinicians assess psychosocial factors, also referred to as "yellow flags" (**Table 7**), in order to appropriately counsel, reassure, and address factors that indicate a poor prognosis and may lead to the development of chronic LBP and long-term disability.[13] It is recommended that this be completed early in the evaluation of back pain, at either the first or second visit. Validated tools, such as STarT Back and Orebro, can be used to assess these psychosocial factors, although there is limited evidence on their ability to prevent disability when interventions are targeted toward their findings[17] (**Table 8**).[25]

In addition, Wadell signs, as outlined in **Table 9**, can be identified during physical examination in order to further guide prognostic outcomes of chronic LBP, but are not validated to predict future disability related to chronic LBP.[26]

Case Discussion

Our patient's historical findings are consistent with radicular pain, possibly related to spinal stenosis, as evidenced by her pseudo-claudication and previous radiographic imaging with disc narrowing. Her history and review of systems do not reveal any red flags, but her social history has several yellow flags, including depression, fear avoidance, and baseline functional impairment, which are important to take note of before determining the best management. This is a recurrent presentation of LBP, but it is of the same characteristic and cause as previous episodes without progressive neurologic deficits, making the need for repeat imaging unnecessary at the time of her presentation.

Treatment regimens offered should prioritize nonpharmacologic therapies, with adjunct pharmacologic therapies if needed. Even in cases of recurrent, acute on chronic LBP, it is likely that her acute symptoms will resolve; thus, she should be counseled as such. Nonpharmacologic therapies should be tailored to her ability to both access and afford, along with personal preference and incorporation of mind-body–based therapies given her psychosocial yellow flags. Therapies that may be ideal here include multidisciplinary rehabilitation, mindfulness-based stress reduction, progressive relaxation, acupuncture, yoga, tai chi, and exercise therapies. If needed, NSAIDs can be used with caution given her history of chronic kidney disease, and hypertension. Although commonly used in clinical practice, evidence does not exist to support the use of anticonvulsants for her radicular pain. If her pain persists, second-line therapies, such as duloxetine, would be a favorable option, especially in the setting of her depression.

Following 6 weeks of management, she should be reevaluated for improvement. If symptoms persist, MRI could be pursued, along with referral to a pain specialist for

Table 7
Comparisons of systemic pharmacologic treatments and their use in acute and chronic low back pain with reduction in pain, disability, and associated harm as rated by quality of evidence

Therapy Type	Magnitude of Pain Reduction	Magnitude of Functional Improvement	Harm Associated with Treatment	Quality of Evidence
Tramadol	**	**	Increased nausea, dizziness, constipation, vomiting, somnolence, dry mouth	Moderate
Duloxetine	*	**	Increased risk for withdrawal due to adverse events, but none serious	Moderate
Opioids	*	*	As noted in **Table 5**	Moderate
NSAIDs	*	*	As noted in **Table 5**	Moderate-low
TCAs	—	—	Not studied	Moderate-low
SSRIs	—	No evidence	Increased risk of adverse events	Moderate
SMRs	Unable to estimate	No evidence	As noted in **Table 5**	Insufficient
Gabapentin/pregabalin	Unable to estimate	Unable to estimate	No clear adverse events	Insufficient
Acetaminophen	No evidence	No evidence	None	

*** high; ** moderate; * small; —, no effect.
Abbreviation: TCA's, tricyclic antidepressants.

Table 8
The Keele STarT back prognostic screening tool

Patient Questions	Responses and Scoring
1. My back pain has spread down my legs at some time in last 2 wk	Agree (1)
2. Pain in shoulder or neck at some time in last 2 wk	Disagree (0)
3. Ability to walk only short distances because of back pain	
4. Dressing more slowly than usual because of back pain	
5. It's not really safe for a person with a condition like mine to be physically active	
6. Worrying thoughts have been going through my mind a lot of the time	
7. I feel that my back pain is terrible and it's never going to get any better	
8. In general I have not enjoyed all the things I used to enjoy	
9. Overall, how bothersome has your back pain been in the last 2 wk?	Not at all (0) Slightly (0) Moderately (0) Very much (1) Extremely (1)
	Total (Q1–9):
Scoring	Subscore (Q5–9):
High risk: subscore 4–5; low risk: total score 0–3; medium risk: all other scores	

From Hill, JC, Whitehurst DG, et al. (2011) Comparison of Stratified Primary Care Management for Low Back Pain with Current Best Practice (STarT Back): a randomized controlled trial. Lancet, 378 (9802), 1560-1571. Reprinted with permission from Elsevier.

Table 9
Psychosocial factors ("yellow flags") and likelihood of predicting long-term disability related to chronic low back pain

Psychosocial Factors (Yellow Flags)	Wadell Physical Examination Findings:
• Belief that pain and activity are harmful (fear avoidance) (+LR 2.5)	• Superficial or nonanatomic tenderness
• Pain somatization (+LR 3.0)	• Nonreproducibility of pain with distraction
• Psychiatric comorbidities/maladaptive coping/catastrophizing (+LR 2.2)	• Regional weakness or sensory change
• Baseline functional impairment (+LR 2.1)	• Overreaction or exaggerated pain response
• Higher physical work demands (+LR 1.4)	
• Lack of work satisfaction (+LR 1.5)	
• Already on/seeking disability compensation (+LR 1.4)	
• Demographic factors (age, sex, race, education, smoking, weight, history of previous back pain) (+LR 0.84–1.3)	
• Prior episodes of LBP (+LR 1.1)	

consideration of epidural steroid injections. In the long term, the patient should be counseled that epidural injections may have only short but immediate benefits. In addition, pursuing surgical intervention would likely not improve her pain unless she began to experience more significant neurologic deficits. At every intervention along the cascade, ongoing patient counseling and education regarding expected outcomes should be discussed in order to set pain and function–related expectations for the patient and prevent setting of goals aimed at complete alleviation of pain and return to baseline function.

CLINICS CARE POINTS

- Evaluating historical and physical examination red flags is key to guiding further workup.
- Evaluating psychosocial yellow flags helps determine prognosis and possibly prevent disability. Tools, such as the STaRT Back prognostic tool, can help focus psychosocial evaluation.
- Diagnostic workup and imaging should focus on high-value, low-cost, low-harm care. Early imaging will rarely change management and often reveals asymptomatic pathologic condition.
- Most episodes of acute and acute on chronic LBP resolve. Initial management should focus on reassurance, education, and avoidance of rest.
- Treatment of LBP often results in only small to moderate reduction in pain and improvement in function. Treatments chosen should be patient-centered, low cost, and low harm.
- Of the nonpharmacologic treatment options, it is best to choose multiple in adjunct, focusing on patient accessibility and preference, with a goal to address psychological factors in patients with psychosocial "yellow" flags.
- Pharmacologic therapies should be used in adjunct or after suboptimal reduction in pain with nonpharmacologic options, but never as solo or first-line therapy. Acetaminophen is no longer recommended as a first-line therapy. SMRs should be considered in treatment of acute LBP and duloxetine as second-line therapy for chronic LBP. Mild opioids, such as tramadol, may be useful in chronic LBP, but should be used in severe, refractory pain.
- Invasive and interventional methods should only be considered in cases of severe LBP that does not respond other treatments, usually after greater than 3 months to 2 years. Epidural steroid injections should not be used routinely for nonradicular chronic LBP.
- Long-term disability can be difficult to predict but can be costly as a result of repeat imaging, outpatient office visits, invasive interventions, and lost workdays.

DISCLOSURE

The authors have nothing to disclose.

REFERENCES

1. Deyo RA, Mirza SK, Martin BI. Back pain prevalence and visit rates. Spine 2006; 31(23):2724–7.

2. Luo X, Pietrobon R, Sun SX, et al. Estimates and patterns of direct health care expenditures among individuals with back pain in the United States. Spine 2003; 29(1):79–86.

3. Chou R, Qaseem A, Snow V, et al. Diagnosis and treatment of low back pain: a joint clinical practice guideline from the American College of Physicians and the American Pain Society. Ann Intern Med 2007;147(7):478–91.
4. Stanton T, Latimer J, Maher C, et al. How do we define the condition 'recurrent low back pain'? A systematic review. Eur Spine J 2010;19(4):533–9.
5. Jarvik JG, Gold LS, Comstock BA, et al. Association of early imaging for back pain with clinical outcomes in older adults. JAMA 2015;313(11):1143–53.
6. Von Korff M, Saunders K. The course of back pain in primary care. Spine 1996; 21(24):2833–7.
7. Deyo R, Mirza S. Herniated lumbar intervertebral disk. N Engl J Med 2016; 374(18):1763–72.
8. Katz J, Harris M. Lumbar spinal stenosis. N Engl J Med 2008;358(8):818–25.
9. Ensrud K, Schousboe J. Vertebral fractures. N Engl J Med 2011;364(17): 1634–42.
10. Zimmerli W. Vertebral osteomyelitis. N Engl J Med 2010;362(11):1022–9.
11. Nagashima H, Tanishima S, Tanida A. Diagnosis and management of spinal infections. J Orthop Sci 2018;23(1):8–13.
12. Patel N, Broderick D, Burns J, et al. ACR appropriateness criteria low back pain. J Am Coll Radiol 2016;13(9):1069–78.
13. Oliveira C, Maher C, Pinto R, et al. Clinical practice guidelines for the management of non-specific low back pain in primary care: an updated overview. Eur Spine J 2018;27(11):2791–803.
14. Chou R, Qaseem A, Owens D, et al. Diagnostic imaging for low back pain: advice for high-value health care from the American College of Physicians. Ann Intern Med 2011;154(3):181–9.
15. Humphreys S, Eck J, Hodges S. Neuroimaging in low back pain. Am Fam Physician 2002;65(11):2299–306.
16. Daffner R, Hackney D. ACR appropriateness criteria on suspected spine trauma. J Am Coll Radiol 2007;4(11):762–75.
17. Last A, Hulbert K. Chronic low back pain: evaluation and management. Am Fam Physician 2009;79(12):1067–74.
18. Qaseem A, Wilt T, McLean R, et al. Noninvasive treatments for acute, subacute, and chronic low back pain: a clinical practice guideline from the American College of Physicians. Ann Intern Med 2017;166(7):514–30.
19. Qin J, Zhang Y, Wu L, et al. Effect of tai chi alone or as additional therapy on low back pain: systematic review and meta-analysis of randomized controlled trials. Medicine 2019;98(37):e17099.
20. Chou R, Deyo R, Friedly J, et al. Nonpharmacologic therapies for low back pain: a systematic review for an American College of Physicians Clinical Practice Guideline. Ann Intern Med 2017;166(7):493–505.
21. Chou R, Friedly J, Skelly A, et al. Systemic pharmacologic therapies for low back pain: a systematic review for an American College of Physicians Clinical Practice Guideline. Ann Intern Med 2017;166(7):480–92.
22. Derry S, Wiffen P, Kalso E, et al. Topical analgesics for acute and chronic pain in adults- an overview of Cochrane Reviews. Cochrane Database Syst Rev 2017;(5):CD008609.
23. Chou R, Hashimoto R, Friedly J, et al. Epidural corticosteroid injections for radiculopathy and spinal stenosis: a systematic review and meta-analysis. Ann Intern Med 2015;163(5):373–81.

24. van Tulder M, Koes B, Seitsalo S, et al. Outcome of invasive treatment modalities on back pain and sciatica: an evidence-based review. Eur Spine J 2006;15(Suppl 1):S82–92.
25. Hill JC, Whitehurst DG, Lewis M, et al. Comparison of stratified primary care management for low back pain with current best practice (STarT Back): a randomized controlled trial. Lancet 2011;378(9802):1560–71.
26. Low Back Pain, Disabling. In: Simel DL, Rennie D. eds. The Rational Clinical Examination: Evidence-Based Clinical Diagnosis. McGraw-Hill; Availablt at: https://jamaevidence-mhmedical-com.proxy.library.emory.edu/content.aspx?bookid=845&sectionid=61357665. Accessed September 30, 2020.

Update on Indigestion

Alia Chisty, MS, MD

KEYWORDS

- Dyspepsia • Functional dyspepsia • Post-prandial distress syndrome
- Epigastric pain syndrome • *Helicobacter pylori* test and treat

KEY POINTS

- Dyspepsia is a complex disorder with high personal and economic cost and incompletely understood pathophysiology that may involve genetic predisposition, gut hypersensitivity, concomitant presence of mood disorders, and disordered pain processing.
- Younger patients less than 60 years old with dyspepsia should not routinely undergo endoscopy.
- For patients with dyspepsia, *H pylori* test-and-treat approach should be taken as the first step followed by proton pump inhibitors.
- For patients with functional dyspepsia, *H pylori* eradication, PPI, TCA, and prokinetic agents should be considered in sequence. Psychotherapy can also be offered to patients, especially those who have underlying mental health conditions.

INTRODUCTION

Indigestion, or dyspepsia, is a common symptom experienced by patients seeking care from their primary care physicians. According to the National Institute of Diabetes and Digestive and Kidney Diseases, indigestion is considered a general term that encompasses a group of gastrointestinal (GI) symptoms that occur together, such as epigastric pain or burning, early satiety, and/or post-prandial discomfort.[1] Up to 30% of the general population in the United States, Canada, and the United Kingdom experience dyspepsia.[2] In the United States alone, dyspepsia costs the health care system about $18 billion per year[3] with even greater societal costs because of missed work or reduced efficacy at work.[4] Patients with dyspepsia experience distress from their symptoms, a perceived reduction in quality of life, and increased economic burden from lost work productivity and medical costs.[2,5,6] Female gender, smoking, using nonsteroidal anti-inflammatory drugs, and positive *Helicobacter pylori* testing are recognized risk factors for dyspepsia.[7]

As per the Rome IV criteria[5] (**Fig. 1**) and the American College of Gastroenterology (ACG) and the Canadian Association of Gastroenterology (CAG) Clinical Guidelines on

Division of General Internal Medicine, Penn State College of Medicine, Penn State Health Milton S. Hershey Medical Center, 500 University Drive, PO Box 850, Hershey, PA 17033, USA
E-mail address: achisty@pennstatehealth.psu.edu

Med Clin N Am 105 (2021) 19–30
https://doi.org/10.1016/j.mcna.2020.08.012
0025-7125/21/© 2020 Elsevier Inc. All rights reserved.

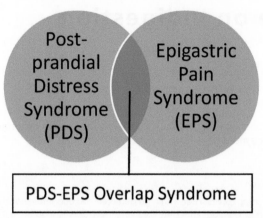

Fig. 1. Functional dyspepsia schematic describing relationship between post-prandial distress syndrome, epigastric pain syndrome, and overlap syndrome.

the Management of Dyspepsia,[8] dyspepsia is predominantly an epigastric pain syndrome (EPS) that lasts for at least 1 month duration and includes such symptoms as epigastric fullness, nausea, vomiting, or heartburn.[8] Dyspepsia caused by an organic, systemic, or metabolic cause discovered through diagnostic evaluation is referred to as secondary dyspepsia.[5] The most common underlying cause is *H pylori* infection, and its treatment leads to symptom improvement or resolution.[5] Approximately 70% of patients with dyspepsia do not have an identifiable organic, systemic, or metabolic cause.[3] Therefore, functional dyspepsia (FD) is characterized by epigastric pain for 1 month for which no organic disease is found on endoscopy.[8]

The Rome IV criteria define FD as one or more symptom of post-prandial discomfort, early satiety, epigastric pain, and epigastric burning that occur at least 3 days per week over 3 months with symptom onset of 6 months.[5,9] Symptoms severity usually disrupts patients' typical activities.[9] FD is an umbrella term that comprises three syndromes: (1) post-prandial distress syndrome (PDS), (2) EPS, and (3) overlapping PDS and EPS (**Table 1**). PDS is characterized by meal-induced dyspeptic symptoms suggesting motility disturbance. It is diagnosed when a patient has bothersome post-prandial fullness and/or bothersome early satiation at least 3 days per week.[5] EPS, however, denotes any epigastric pain or burning that can occur during fasting or after

Table 1	
Rome IV diagnostic criteria for functional dyspepsia	
Presence of ≥1 of the following symptoms for past 3 mo with symptom onset ≥6 mo before diagnosis:	
• Bothersome post-prandial fullness	≥3 d per wk
• Bothersome early satiety	≥3 d per wk
• Bothersome epigastric pain	≥1 d per wk
• Bothersome epigastric burning	≥1 d per wk
Must also have:	
No evidence of structure disease on esophagogastroduodenoscopy or other organic, systemic, or metabolic explanation for symptoms	

Data from Stanghellini V, Chan FKL, Hasler WL, Malagelada JR, Suzuki H, Tack J, Talley NJ. Gastroduodenal Disorders. Gastroenterology 2016;150:1380-1392.

meal ingestion. It is diagnosed by bothersome epigastric pain and/or burning for at least 1 day a week (**Table 2**).[5]

PDS-EPS overlap syndrome characterizes discomfort following meal ingestion and epigastric symptoms of pain or burning (see **Fig. 1**).[9] Vomiting, symptoms of gastro-esophageal reflux, biliary pain, and symptoms of peptic ulcer disease and should be distinguished from PDS and EPS because symptoms can overlap. Patients with FD rarely report frequent vomiting. This symptom should trigger further diagnostic investigation.[5]

PATHOPHYSIOLOGY

Causes of dyspepsia are multifactorial. When an underlying condition, such as *H pylori* infection, is identified and eradicated, symptoms can improve.[8,10] However, functional GI disorders point toward disordered interaction between the gut and the brain.[11] The pathophysiology of FD is not completely explained. Motor and sensory dysfunction of the gastroduodenal structure, compromised mucosal integrity, immune activation, and dysregulation of the gut-brain axis are thought to play a role in explaining symptoms.[12]

Infection with *H pylori* results in chronic mucosal inflammation in the stomach and duodenum, which might lead to GI sensitivity and motility dysfunction. Chronic inflammation and gastritis can affect endocrine functions of the stomach, such as the production of somatostatin, gastrin, and ghrelin. Further studies are required to confirm this hypothesis.[10] From a Cochrane review from 2005, *H pylori* eradication in nonulcerative disease showed a statistically significant relative risk (RR) reduction of 9% on long-term symptom relief when compared with placebo in all subtypes of FD.[13] The efficacy of eradication therapy was more prominent in patients of Asian descent.[10,13]

It is estimated that delayed gastric emptying can occur in about 25% to 35% of patients with FD.[14] Furthermore, it has been observed that 30% to 40% of patients experience a reduced gastric relaxation response to food ingestion and decreased fundic accommodation, especially in postinfection dyspepsia.[5,15,16] Hypersensitivity to chemical stimuli, such as intraluminal acids and lipids,[17] duodenal eosinophilia related to early satiety,[18] and acute GI infection[19] can trigger resultant symptoms of FD. Mental health disorders, specifically anxiety and depression, have been shown to be associated with FD.[20] Physical and emotional abuse in adulthood may also play a role.[5,20] It has been proposed that in certain genetically predisposed patients,

Table 2 Defining PDS and EPS	
Post-prandial Distress Syndrome	**Epigastric Pain Syndrome**
Presence of ≥1 of the following symptoms ≥3 d per wk:	Presence of ≥1 of the following symptoms ≥1 d per wk:
Bothersome post-prandial fullness	Bothersome epigastric pain
Bothersome early satiety	Bothersome epigastric burning
Must also have:	
No evidence of structure disease on esophagogastroduodenoscopy or other organic, systemic, or metabolic explanation for symptoms	
Criteria fulfilled for past 3 mo with symptom onset ≥6 mo before diagnosis	

Data from Stanghellini V, Chan FKL, Hasler WL, Malagelada JR, Suzuki H, Tack J, Talley NJ. Gastroduodenal Disorders. Gastroenterology 2016;150:1380-1392.

certain allergens or infections can trigger barrier disruption, immune activation, T2 helper cell response, and eosinophil-induced degranulation that can lead to tissue injury or healing in the gut.[21] If the duodenum becomes inflamed in this process, it is postulated to be sensitive to acid and can cause cytokine release that would result in meal-related discomfort.[21]

DIFFERENTIAL DIAGNOSIS

The differential diagnosis for dyspepsia is broad and includes abdominal, chest, or iatrogenic reasons for discomfort and disease. The main imitators include gastroesophageal reflux disease (GERD), esophagitis, esophageal malignancy, gastric or duodenal peptic ulcer disease, gastric malignancy, hepatitis, hepatic malignancy cholelithiasis, cholecystitis, pancreatitis, pancreatic malignancy, ischemic heart disease, mesenteric ischemia, or iatrogenic from certain medications.[22] The medications that are often cited as causing dyspepsia include: nonsteroidal anti-inflammatory drugs, aspirin, steroids, certain antibiotics, bisphosphonates, serotonin-norepinephrine receptor inhibitors, theophylline, and calcium channel blockers.[22] Therefore, it is critical to obtain a thorough history when evaluating patients with dyspepsia with attention paid to medication use, including over-the-counter medications.

EVALUATION

Primary care physicians should first obtain a thorough history including assessing for risk factors for GI malignancy; iatrogenic or medication-related causes of dyspepsia; risk for *H pylori* infection; and assessment for common concurrent conditions, such as GERD and irritable bowel disease.[14] Gastric cancer, which can present with dyspepsia, is recognized to be the third most common cause of global cancer mortality and represents about 8.2% of cancer-related deaths from 2018.[23] In 2017, the ACG and the CAG published their joint guidelines on dyspepsia, which increased the age from 55 to 60 for evaluation with esophagogastroduodenoscopy for patients presenting with new dyspepsia of unknown cause.[8] However, they also recommend that for patients from South East Asia and some South American countries with higher risk of GI malignancy, physicians should use their clinical judgment to guide their decision to obtain an endoscopy at a younger age.[8] GI malignancy is found to be two-fold higher in men than women when adjusted for age.[8] Therefore, sex should be considered in borderline cases.

For patients younger than age 60 who have dyspepsia along with alarm features, such as weight loss, anemia, dysphagia, and persistent vomiting, it is no longer recommended to obtain an esophagogastroduodenoscopy to exclude upper GI malignancy.[8] Individual alarm features do carry about a two to three times increased risk of malignancy, but usually these are seen with older patients.[8] Multiple studies show that alarm features have a low positive predictive value and are of limited value in stratifying patients for endoscopy[24–27] in patients who present with dyspepsia.[8] This recommendation is based on moderate quality data and the need for endoscopy should be taken in a case-by-case basis.

For patients younger than the age of 60, the ACG and CAG recommend that patients should undergo noninvasive testing for *H pylori* and be treated accordingly if positive.[8] This is a strong recommendation based on high-quality evidence. This test-and-treat strategy is superior from diagnostic and cost-effective perspectives.[28] The preferred testing methods include 13C urea breath test or the fecal monoclonal antigen test, both of which have high sensitivity and specificity for active *H pylori* infection when compared with biopsies.[28,29] Urea breath test may require a referral to a gastroenterologist and is not easy to perform by a primary care physician. In comparison, fecal monoclonal antigen test is easy to order and is performed without requiring any referrals or invasive procedures making it easy to obtain in the primary care setting. Serum antibody testing is not preferred because it can remain positive for several years even after H pylori infection has been successfully eradicated.[8,29]

TREATMENT
Treatment Recommendations for Undiagnosed Dyspepsia

For patients who were H pylori negative or continued to have dyspeptic symptoms after H pylori eradication, those patients should be started on empiric acid-suppression therapy with a proton pump inhibitor (PPI).[8] This recommendation is based on high-quality evidence. If patients do not respond to PPIs, then a prokinetic agent should be tried. There are little, low-quality data on evaluating prokinetic therapy in the treatment of undiagnosed dyspepsia. Prokinetic agents have a high side effect profile, are not readily available, and should be used at the lowest effective dose. In the United States, metoclopramide should not be used for more than 12 weeks and domperidone dose should not exceed 30 mg daily.[8]

For patients younger than 60 years old with undiagnosed dyspepsia, who have received H pylori eradication and not responding to PPI treatment, tricyclic antidepressants (TCAs) are offered as a treatment choice.[8] This recommendation is extrapolated from a systematic review and meta-analysis study involving patients with FD and found that patients treated with a TCA or an antipsychotic medication had a decrease in symptoms with a number needed to treat (NNT) of six (95% confidence interval [CI], 4–16) when compared with placebo.[30]

Treatment of Functional Dyspepsia

Eradications of Helicobacter pylori
Eradication of H pylori in patients with FD may be beneficial and should be a shared decision between the patient and the physician. A systematic review and meta-analysis including 25 randomized controlled trials (RCTs) including 5555 patients with FD suggests that H pylori eradication therapy is beneficial for long-term symptom relief but does not have short-term benefits. Additionally, it can reduce the development of peptic ulceration and lead to histologic resolution of chronic gastritis. Despite these benefits, eradication does not seem to improve quality of life, and patients may experience adverse medication effects from treatment.[31]

In an earlier meta-analysis, dyspepsia symptoms significantly improved in European (odds ratio, 1.49; 95% CI, 1.10–2.02), Asian (odds ratio, 1.54; 95% CI, 1.07–2.21), and US (odds ratio, 1.43; 95% CI, 1.12–1.83) populations when comparing H pylori eradication with control groups.[32] This may suggest that if the decision to treat is made, treatment of underlying H pylori can be effective for addressing symptoms of FD across various populations.[32] Furthermore, patients with FD and concomitant H pylori infection with microscopic duodenitis may experience more severe symptoms.[33] In a prospective trial of 37 patients in Iran, patients with both microscopic duodenitis and H pylori infection had initially higher scores on the validated Leeds dyspepsia questionnaire and experienced a significantly greater decrease in symptoms at 3 and 6 months, respectively, when compared with patients with H pylori without microscopic duodenitis.[34] When considering which patients with FD might benefit from H pylori eradication, physicians could improve severity of FD symptoms if H pylori is eliminated in patients with underlying microscopic duodenitis.

Proton pump inhibitors

The ACG/CAG clinical guidelines on the management of dyspepsia recommend initiating PPI therapy for patients with FD who continue to have symptoms despite *H pylori* eradication or absence,[8] a recommendation based on moderate-quality data. A Cochrane review in 2017 identified 23 RCTs including 8759 participants to study the effect of PPIs on quality of life symptom improvement when compared directly with placebo, with H_2-receptor antagonists, or with prokinetic medications.[35]

In patients with FD, 2 to 8 weeks of PPI therapy improved symptoms of dyspepsia when compared with placebo (RR, 0.88; 95% CI, 0.82–0.94), when compared with H_2-blockers (RR, 0.8; 95% CI, 0.74–1.04), and when compared with prokinetic agents (RR, 0.90; 95% CI, 0.81–1.00).[35] The quality of evidence ranged from moderate for the PPI studies against placebo but dropped to low quality against H_2-blockers and prokinetic agents.[35] There are moderate-quality data that PPIs when used in conjunction with prokinetic medications offered patients a higher benefit than PPIs alone in reducing symptoms of dyspepsia in patients with FD (RR, 0.85; 95% CI, 0.68–1.08).[35] The NNT ranged from 13 to 20 in these grouped analyses.[35]

PPIs should be considered as a readily available, reasonably tolerated, and somewhat effective treatment of FD when compared with placebo. This benefit persists despite low or standard dose of PPI and independent of duration of treatment.[35] Therefore, for patients with FD who continue to have symptoms despite *H pylori* eradiation or without *H pylori* infection, PPI therapy should be considered.

Tricyclic antidepressants

Because patients with FD exhibit signs of abnormal pain processing, hypersensitivity of the viscera, and depressed mood or anxiety, researchers have examined the efficacy of psychotropic medications in the treatment of FD. In a systematic review and meta-analysis by Lu and colleagues,[36] eight RCTs were pooled to find an RR of 0.76 (95% CI, 0.62–0.94; $P = .01$) of TCAs compared with placebo, illustrating an improvement in symptoms on TCAs. This same study did not find any benefit of selective serotonin reuptake inhibitors; however, when compared with placebo, patients experienced adverse events more frequently on antidepressants (RR, 1.64; 95% CI, 1.14–2.35; $P = .007$). In a subsequent systematic review and meta-analysis by Ford and colleagues[30] involving 13 RCTs with 1241 patients, antipsychotic agents and TCAs demonstrated benefit when compared with placebo, with an RR of 0.78 (95% CI, 0.68–0.91) and NNT of six (95% CI, 4–16), but did not extend to selective serotonin reuptake inhibitors. Patients on psychotropic medications, however, experienced greater adverse events, including those that led to withdrawal of the medications, with a number needed to harm of 21 for TCAs and antipsychotic medications.[30]

Based on moderate-quality evidence, the ACG/CAG guidelines recommend TCAs for treatment of patients who do not respond to PPI or *H pylori* eradication.[8] Following this recommendation, a single-center, double-blind, RCT of *H pylori*–negative patients compared imipramine with placebo for 12 weeks in patients who had refractory symptoms of FD after PPI and domperidone use.[37] This study confirmed that TCAs can benefit patients with FD. Relief of global dyspepsia symptoms at 12 weeks occurred in 63.6% (95% CI, 50.4–75.1) of patients on imipramine when compared with placebo (36.5%; 95% CI, 24.8–50.1; $P = .0051$).[37] However, a greater percentage of patients on imipramine had to discontinue use because of side effects (18% in TCA group, 8% in placebo).[37] Therefore, especially in refractory FD, TCAs should be considered as a possible therapy but patients should be adequately counseled as to potential side effects and should engage in a shared decision between physicians and patients.

Prokinetic therapy
At the time of the ACG/CAG joint guidelines, many of the studies involving prokinetic agents included such medications as cisapride, domperidone, and metoclopramide. Because of safety concerns, cisapride has been removed from the US market; domperidone is not readily available and needs to be approved on a case-by-case basis for use by the Food and Drug Administration[38]; and metoclopramide is not meant for long-term use because of side effects of dystonia, Parkinson-like movements, and tardive dyskinesis. Because of low-quality data and high risk of bias in studies involving prokinetic agents and high risk of adverse events of these medications, the ACG/CAG guidelines recommend prokinetic therapy after patients fail to respond to *H pylori* eradication, PPI use, or TCA therapy.[8]

Following these guidelines, a systematic review and meta-analysis of RCTs involving prokinetic agents was published by Pittayanon and colleagues[39] in 2019 that reviewed 38 studies. Regardless of FD subtype, prokinetic agents reduced global symptoms of FD (RR, 0.81 [95% CI, 0.74–0.89]; NNT, 7 [95% CI, 5–12]). Even after removing the data for cisapride, global symptom improvement for prokinetic agents remained significant (RR, 0.87 [95% CI, 0.80–0.94]; $P = .0004$; NNT, 12 [95% CI, 8–27]).[39] Nine of these trials directly compared two prokinetic agents, and domperidone 10 mg was most often used as a comparator.[39] No major differences between prokinetic agents were found.[39] Unfortunately, no difference was found in quality of life scores between patients in the prokinetic group compared with placebo in pooled data involving 1774 patients and no difference in adverse events when comparing prokinetic agents (29.3%) with placebo (30.8%).[39] When comparing prokinetic agents and adverse events, only cisapride (RR, 1.31; 95% CI, 1.03–1.65; $P = .03$) had greater adverse effects in the active treatment group with a number needed to harm of 23.[39] This systematic review suggests that prokinetics may be effective in the treatment of FD without differences between prokinetic agents; however, the quality of the data remains low.[39] Higher quality RCTs are required to ascertain the actual benefit of prokinetic agents in FD treatment.

Psychological therapies
Psychological factors play an important role in functional GI disorders with strong associations between depression and anxiety with FD. From a review of 12 RCTs involving 1563 patients with FD, all 12 trials found a significant benefit of psychological therapies when compared with usual care.[8] In these studies, a variety of therapies were offered, but cognitive behavioral therapy was most commonly used.[8] Despite the impressive positive finding, it should be noted that these studies were low quality with a high risk of bias and no blinding.[8] The ACG/CAG guidelines recommend psychological therapies as a conditional recommendation because of the quality of the data, the high degree of patient motivation required, and potentially high cost to the patient.[8] There is a growing body of literature to support the biopsychosocial framework for the development and manifestation of functional GI disorders, with multiple studies evaluating irritable bowel syndrome and FD.[40] In this model, it is essential to consider and address environmental, psychological, and biologic factors for appropriate treatment of functional GI disorders.[40] Therefore, higher quality studies are required to better ascertain the effects of psychological therapy on the treatment of FD.

Alternative treatments
The ACG/CAG guidelines recommend against use of complementary or alternative medicines for FD.[8] There are numerous proposed alternative supplements that have

been studied, but the studies are too diverse, are of poor methodologic quality, or it is unclear if the benefit is clinically significant for any conclusion to be drawn.[8] Some herbal supplements, such as iberogast (STW5), a blend of nine different herbs including angelica, bitter candy-fruit, caraway, celandine, chamomile, licorice, Melissa, milk thistle, and peppermint, had limited improvement clinically when compared with placebo.[41] Studies of supplements have variable quality with high heterogeneity.

In a Cochrane Review published in 2014, authors acknowledged that acupuncture and electroacupuncture are commonly used modalities for treatment of FD in Asian countries.[42] However, there are limited data of variable quality that demonstrate if there is any benefit to acupuncture as a noninvasive treatment modality. A total of seven studies were included in the review but had a high risk of bias because of the inability to blind.[42] Four of the trials compared acupuncture with a commonly used pharmacotherapy for FD without clear evidence to its safety and effectiveness when compared with motility agents.[42] Because of the low quality of evidence, it is unclear if acupuncture can benefit patients with FD compared with other treatment modalities.[42]

In a recent small study by Yang and colleagues[43] conducted in China, patients who met Rome IV criteria for PDS were assigned to short sessions of acupuncture or sham acupuncture over 4 weeks. In the acupuncture group, 27.8% of patients experienced elimination of all three cardinal symptoms of PDS compared with 17.3% in the sham acupuncture group and was maintained for up to 12 weeks after treatment.[43] There were several notable limitations, such as high attrition rate, inability to blind acupuncturists, and most importantly, lack of objective outcomes.[43] However, no patients experienced any adverse effects of treatment in either treatment group.[43]

There are insufficient data to support the recommendation of any complementary or alternative treatment modalities for FD. However, for some patients who may request pursing herbal remedies or acupuncture, this should be a shared decision between the physician and the patient and the patient should be counseled that there is insufficient evidence to oppose the use of complementary treatments in FD.

Motility studies

Motility studies are not routinely recommended for patients with FD.[8] However, if there is a strong suspicion that gastroparesis is strongly impacting symptomology, then it should be considered.[8]

Dietary interventions

There are no guideline recommendations to support any dietary modifications in the treatment of FD. There are some studies suggesting associations between ingestion of certain foods and increase symptoms of dyspepsia. A systematic review of 16 studies showed an association between dietary fat, gluten, fermentable oligo-, di-, mono-saccharides, and polyols (FODMAPs); food chemicals, such as chili peppers; and caffeinated beverages, such as tea and coffee were associated with symptoms of FD.[44] There is inconclusive evidence if alcohol consumption leads to symptoms of FD; however, there may be an association with the type of alcohol consumed (beer, wine, liquor).[44] This study illustrates the importance of further investigation of the role of dietary modification in FD and implicates the use of low-risk interventions, such as a FODMAP diet or a gluten-free diet, in ameliorating the symptoms of FD.[45]

Probiotics and prebiotics

In a systematic and meta-analysis of five RCTs that included adult patients with FD and compared prebiotics, probiotics, or synbiotics with either placebo or no specific treatment, of the five eligible studies, four RCTs assessed the efficacy of probiotics for FD and one study included prebiotics encompassing a total of 409 patients.[46] Overall, prebiotics and probiotics improved symptoms of FD with an RR of symptom improvement after treatment to be 1.15 (95% CI, 1.01–1.30) when compared with placebo.[46] There was a trend toward a beneficial effect of probiotics alone, but the results were not statistically significant.[46] No specific strains or species of probiotics were identified.[46] Overall, only two adverse events occurred in the intervention group compared with eight in the placebo group.[46] No trials involving synbiotics were included in the study, and therefore, no specific recommendation for their use can be made.[46] Therefore, with the safety profile, it is reasonable to suggest use of probiotics or prebiotics in the treatment of FD if other evidence-based treatment strategies are not successfully controlling patient's symptoms.

PREGNANCY AND DYSPEPSIA

GERD is a common symptom of pregnancy. A Cochrane review of four trials involved 358 women.[47] Two trials directly compared pharmacologic treatment with placebo, one study included acupuncture, and one study evaluated pharmacologic treatment compared with lifestyle and dietary modification.[47] The group of pregnant women in the intervention group sustained complete resolution of symptoms compared with the women in the placebo or no treatment group with an RR of 1.85 (95% CI, 1.36–2.50) based on moderate-quality evidence from two trials.[47] One study used a medication no longer available (intramuscular prostigmine), compared with the second study, which used a combination of magnesium aluminum hydroxide and simethicone.[47] In one study comparing sucralfate use with diet and lifestyle changes, the medication group experienced complete resolution of symptoms with an RR of 2.41 (95% CI, 1.42–4.07). Finally, acupuncture improved sleeping (RR, 2.80; 95% CI, 1.14–6.86) and eating ability (RR, 2.40; 95% CI, 1.11–5.18) but did not comment on the specific relief from GERD symptoms.[47] This was a small RCT involving only 36 women.[47] More studies are needed to make any definitive recommendations; however, primary care physicians can consider magnesium aluminum hydroxide and simethicone as possible options in providing pregnant women with some GERD relief.

SUMMARY

Indigestion, or dyspepsia, is a commonly seen symptom that can greatly affect the quality of life and productivity of an individual. The 2017 ACG/CAG guidelines recommend that patients younger than 60 not routinely obtain endoscopy because of lower prevalence of gastric cancer at a younger age, but with the caveat that physician judgment should be used to assess individual patient risk based on race/ethnicity (Southeast Asian descent) and/or presence of more than one alarm symptom for malignancy. For patients with undifferentiated dyspepsia, patients should first undergo a test-and-treat approach for *H pylori* followed by PPI use, then prokinetic therapy or TCA use. For patients diagnosed with FD, treatment recommendations still include *H pylori* eradication if detected, followed by PPI, TCA, prokinetic agents, and finally psychotherapy. There is insufficient evidence to support complementary medicine options. Motility studies are not routinely suggested. There is a growing body of literature addressing dietary modification and probiotics in the treatment of FD, both of which are safe and low-risk interventions. Further research is required to integrate dietary modification into guideline-recommended therapy.

CLINICAL CARE POINTS

- Functional dyspepsia is an umbrella term that encompasses three syndromes: post-prandial distress syndrome (PDS), epigastric pain syndrome (EPS), and overlapping PDS and EPS.
- Functional dyspepsia can be diagnosed using the Rome IV diagnostic criteria.
- For patients younger than age 60, Helicobacter pylori test and treat approach should be first line treatment.
- Motility studies are not routinely recommended for patients unless there is a strong suspicion of gastroparesis.
- There is a growing body of evidence to suggest dietary modification and probiotics as treatment options for FD, however, further research is needed to integrate these options into clinical guidelines.

DISCLOSURE

The author has nothing to disclose.

REFERENCES

1. Available at: https://www.niddk.nih.gov/health-information/digestive-diseases/indigestion-dyspepsia/definition-facts (last Accessed May 7, 2020)
2. Lacy BE, Weiser KT, Kennedy AT, et al. Functional dyspepsia: the economic impact to patients. Aliment Pharmacol Ther 2013;38:170–7.
3. Aziz I, Palsson OS, Törnblom H, et al. Epidemiology, clinical characteristics, and associations for symptom-based Rome IV functional dyspepsia in adults in the USA, Canada, and the UK: a cross-sectional population-based study. Lancet Gastroenterol Hepatol 2018;3(4):252–62.
4. Moayyedi P, Mason J. Clinical and economic consequences of dyspepsia in the community. Gut 2002;50(suppl 4):10–2.
5. Stanghellini V, Chan FKL, Hasler WL, et al. Gastroduodenal disorders. Gastroenterology 2016;150:1380–92.
6. Sander GB, Mazzoleni LE, Francesconi CF, et al, Helicobacter Eradication Relief of Dyspetic Symptoms Trial Investigators. Influence of organic and functional dyspepsia on work productivity: the HEROES-DIP study. Value Health 2011; 14(5 Suppl 1):S126–9.
7. Ford AC, Marwaha A, Sood R. , et al. Global prevalence of, and risk factors for, uninvestigated dyspepsia. Gut 2015;64(7):1049–57.
8. Moayyedi PM, Lacy BE, Andrews CN, et al. ACG and CAG clinical guideline: management of dyspepsia. Am J Gastroenterol 2017;112(7):988–1013.
9. Stanghellini V. Functional dyspepsia and irritable bowel syndrome: beyond Rome IV. Dig Dis 2017;35:14–7.
10. Suzuki H, Moayyedi P. Helicobacter pylori infection in functional dyspepsia. Nat Rev Gastroenterol Hepatol 2013;10:168–74.
11. Drossman DA. Functional gastrointestinal disorders: history, pathophysiology, clinical features, and Rome IV. Gastroenterology 2016;150:1262–79.
12. Vanheel H, Farre R. Changes in gastrointestinal tract function and structure in functional dyspepsia. Nat Rev Gastroenterol Hepatol 2013;10:142–9.
13. Moayyedi P, Soo S, Deeks J, et al. Eradication of Helicobacter pylori for non-ulcer dyspepsia. Cochrane Database Syst Rev 2005;(2):CD002096.
14. Stanghellini V, Tack J. Gastroparesis: separate entity or just a part of dyspepsia? Gut 2014;63:972–1978.

15. Tack J, Piessevaux H, Coulie B, et al. Role of impaired gastric accommodation to a meal in functional dyspepsia. Gastroenterology 1998;115:1346–52.
16. Kindt S, Tack J. Impaired gastric accommodation and its role in dyspepsia. Gut 2006;55(12):1685-1691. https://doi.org/10.1136/gut.2005.085365.
17. Bratten J, Jones MP. Prolonged recording of duodenal acid exposure in patients with functional dyspepsia and controls using a radiotelemetry pH monitoring system. J Clin Gastroenterol 2009;43:527–33.
18. Walker MM, Aggarwal KR, Shim LS, et al. Duodenal eosinophilia and dyspepsia. J Gastroenterol Hepatol 2014;29:474–9.
19. Talley NJ. Functional dyspepsia: advances in diagnosis and therapy. Gut Liver 2017;11(3):349-357. https://doi.org/10.5009/gnl16055.
20. Adibi P, Keshteli AH, Daghaghzadeh H, et al. Association of anxiety, depression, and psychological distress in people with and without functional dyspepsia. Adv Biomed Res 2016;5:195.
21. Talley NJ, Ford AC. Functional dyspepsia. N Engl J Med 2015;373:1853–63. https://doi.org/10.1056/NEJMra1501505.
22. Overland MK. Dyspepsia. Med Clin N Am 2014;98:549–64.
23. GLOBCAN project, International Agency for Research on Cancer. World Health Organization. Available at: https://gco.iarc.fr/today/data/factsheets/cancers/39-All-cancers-fact-sheet.pdfb. Accessed May 10, 2020.
24. Vakil N, Moayyedi P, Fennerty MB, et al. Limited value of alarm features in the diagnosis of upper gastrointestinal malignancy: systematic review and meta-analysis. Gastroenterology 2006;131:390–401.
25. Collins GS, Altman DG. Identifying patients with undetected gastro-oesophageal cancer in primary care: external validation of QCancer® (Gastro-Oesophageal). Eur J Cancer 2013;49:1040–8.
26. Jones R, Latinovic R, Charlton J, et al. Alarm symptoms in early diagnosis of cancer in primary care" cohort study using General Practice Research Database. BMJ 2007;334:1040.
27. Stapley S, Peters TJ, Neal RD, et al. The risk of oesophago-gastric cancer in symptomatic patients in primary care: a large case-control study using electronic records. Br J Cancer 2013;108:25–31.
28. Chey WD, Leontiadis GI, Howden CW, et al. ACG clinical guideline: treatment of *Helicobacter pylori* infection. Am J Gastroenterol 2017;112(2):212–39.
29. Malfertheiner P, Venerito M, Schulz C. *Helicobacter pylori* infection: new facts in clinical management. Curr Treat Options Gastro 2018;16:605–15.
30. Ford AC, Luthra P, Tack J, et al. Efficacy of psychotropic drugs in functional dyspepsia: systematic review and meta-analysis. Gut 2017;66:411–20.
31. Du LJ, Chen BR, Kim JJ, et al. *Helicobacter pylori* eradication therapy for functional dyspepsia: systematic review and meta-analysis. World J Gastroenterol 2016;22(12):3486–95. https://doi.org/10.3748/wjg.v22.i12.3486.
32. Zhao B, Zhao J, Cheng WF, Shi WJ, Liu W, Pan XL, Zhang GX. Efficacy of *Helicobacter pylori* eradication therapy on functional dyspepsia: a meta-analysis of randomized controlled studies with 12-month follow-up. J Clin Gastroenterol March 2014;48(3):241–7.
33. Mirbagheri SA, Khajavirad N, Rakhshani N, et al. Impact of *Helicobacter pylori* infection and microscopic duodenal histopathological changes on clinical symptoms of patients with functional dyspepsia. Dig Dis Sci 2012;57:967–72.
34. Mirbagheri SS, Mirbagheri SA, Nabavizadeh B, et al. Impact of microscopic duodenitis on symptomatic response to *Helicobacter pylori* eradication in functional dyspepsia. Dig Dis Sci 2015;60:163–7.

35. Pinto-Sanchez MI, Yuan Y, Bercik P, et al. Proton pump inhibitors for functional dyspepsia. Cochrane Database Syst Rev 2017;(3):CD011194.
36. Lu Y, Chen M, Huang Z, et al. Antidepressants in the treatment of functional dyspepsia: a systematic review and meta-analysis. PLoS One 2016;11(6): e0157798.
37. Cheong PK, Ford AC, Cheung CKY, et al. Low-dose imipramine for refractory functional dyspepsia: a randomised, double-blind, placebo-controlled trial. Lancet Gastroenterol Hepatol 2018;3(12):837–44.
38. Available at: https://www.fda.gov/drugs/investigational-new-drug-ind-application/ how-request-domperidone-expanded-access-use last Accessed May 22, 2020
39. Pittayanon R, Yuan Y, Bollegala NP, et al. Prokinetics for functional dyspepsia. Am J Gastroenterol 2019;114:233–43. https://doi.org/10.1038/s41395-018-0258-6.
40. Van Oudenhove L, Levy RL, Crowell MD, et al. Biopsychosocial aspects of functional gastrointestinal disorders: how central and environmental processes contribute to the development and expression of functional gastrointestinal disorders. Gastroenterology 2016;150:1355–67.
41. Von Arnim U, Peitz U, Vinson B, et al. STW 5, a phytopharmacon for patients with functional dyspepsia: results of a multicenter, placebo-controlled double-blind study. Am J Gastroenterol 2007;102(6):1268–75.
42. Lan L, Zeng F, Liu GJ, et al. Acupuncture for functional dyspepsia. Cochrane Database Syst Rev 2014;(10):CD008487.
43. Yang JW, Wang LQ, Zou X, et al. Effect of acupuncture for postprandial distress syndrome: a randomized clinical trial. Ann Intern Med 2020;172(12):777–85.
44. Duncanson KR, Talley NJ, Walker MM, et al. Food and functional dyspepsia: a systematic review. J Hum Nutr Diet 2018;31:390–407.
45. Mounsey A, Barzin A, Rietz A. Functional dyspepsia: evaluation and management. Am Fam Physician 2020;101(2):84–8.
46. Zhang J, Wu HM, Wang X, et al. Efficacy of prebiotics and probiotics for functional dyspepsia: a systematic review and meta-analysis. Medicine (Baltimore) 2020;99(7):e19107.
47. Phupong V, Hanprasertpong T. Interventions for heartburn in pregnancy. Cochrane Database Syst Rev 2015;(9):CD011379.

Approach to the Patient with Cough

Joshua A. Davis, MD[a], Kirana Gudi, MD[b],*

KEYWORDS

- Approach to cough • Chronic cough • Cough in the primary care setting
- Algorithm for treatment of cough

KEY POINTS

- The duration of the symptom divides cough into acute (less than 3 weeks), subacute (3–8 weeks), and chronic (greater than 8 weeks); the duration often has diagnostic implications so a careful history is key.
- Acute cough is most commonly caused by acute respiratory infections of the upper and lower airways.
- The initial evaluation for the patient with chronic cough is much reliant on a thorough history and physical examination.

INTRODUCTION

Cough is one of the most common reasons a patient may seek care in the outpatient setting, and leads to approximately 30 million clinical encounters per year in the United States alone.[1] Cough has also been observed to prompt nearly 40% of office visits to a pulmonologist.[2] The approach to this common and troubling symptom is discussed.

CLASSIFICATION OF COUGH

The duration of the symptom divides cough into acute (less than 3 weeks), subacute (3–8 weeks), and chronic (greater than 8 weeks); the duration often has diagnostic implications so a careful history is key. Respiratory infections are the most common cause for acute cough and may be implicated in an acute exacerbation of a chronic lung disease (eg, chronic obstructive pulmonary disease). Pulmonary embolism has rarely been noted to cause cough and should be considered if other elements of the history, signs, and symptoms rouse suspicion.[3]

[a] Division of Pulmonary and Critical Care Medicine, New York-Presbyterian Hospital, Weill Cornell Campus, New York, NY, USA; [b] Weill Department of Medicine, Weill Cornell Medicine, 525 East 68th Street, New York, NY 10065, USA
* Corresponding author.
E-mail address: kig2001@med.cornell.edu

Med Clin N Am 105 (2021) 31–38
https://doi.org/10.1016/j.mcna.2020.08.013
0025-7125/21/© 2020 Elsevier Inc. All rights reserved.

PATHOPHYSIOLOGY OF COUGH

Stimulation of a cough receptor initiates the cough reflex arc. Cough receptors are divided into those found in the respiratory tract and those outside of the respiratory tract. Extrarespiratory cough receptors are found within adjacent structures, such as the pericardium, esophagus, diaphragm, stomach, auditory canal, and tympanic membranes. Cough receptors are further divided into those whose reflex arc is initiated by mechanical or chemical stimuli. Chemical cough receptors are found within and outside of the respiratory tract, and are triggered by many different stimuli, which include acid, cold, heat, capsaicin/capsaicin-like compounds, and fragrances. Mechanical receptors, which are triggered by touch or displacement, typically from inhaled particulate matter, are located solely within the larynx and tracheobronchial tree. Once stimulated, impulses from cough receptors travel to the cough center in the medulla via the vagus nerve. The cough center, which is also under cortical control, then produces efferent signals via the phrenic nerve, vagus nerve, and spinal motor neurons to the diaphragm, larynx, trachea, and bronchi, and the expiratory muscles and pelvic sphincters, respectively.[4] This coordinated effort produces a violent expulsion of air to protect the gas exchange function of the lungs.

ETIOLOGIES

Acute cough is most commonly caused by acute respiratory infections of the upper and lower airways (**Table 1**). However, when patients lack associated symptoms, such as fever, myalgias, and sore throat, hay fever or allergic rhinitis should be considered. Acute exposure to the inhalation of irritants can also cause acute cough in the right historical context.

Subacute cough, which is cough that lasts between 3 and 8 weeks, has several potential etiologies. Most commonly this follows nonspecific viral infections that have caused inflammation of the airways. Postviral cough usually improves spontaneously, but because of the prolonged symptom, there are many treatments used for alleviation. These include a trail of inhaled ipratropium, inhaled corticosteroids, or perhaps oral steroids.[5]

Bordetella pertussis may be an underrecognized cause of subacute and postinfectious cough. Diagnosis of pertussis requires a high index of suspicion. Cough of 2 weeks' duration and longer, along with coughing paroxysms, inspiratory "whoop," and posttussive emesis may suggest pertussis. These classic manifestations are less likely to be present in patients with prior immunity. Initially, culture and polymerase chain reaction testing from polyester nasopharyngeal swabs may be useful; after

Table 1
Etiologies of cough

Acute	Subacute	Chronic
Upper respiratory tract infections	Postinfectious cough	Upper airway cough syndrome
Lower respiratory tract infections		Gastroesophageal reflux
Hay fever, allergic rhinitis	Pertussis	Asthma
Inhalational exposure	Angiotensin-converting enzyme inhibitors	Angiotensin-converting enzyme inhibitors
		Chronic bronchitis
		Foreign bodies
		Tracheobronchomalacia
		Bronchiectasis
		Lung cancer

4 weeks, only serology is useful. Generally, antibiotics are not indicated 3 weeks beyond onset of symptoms; the cough at this stage is not caused by active infection, but rather local tissue damage.[6] Because of this, from a public health perspective the risk of transmission is decreased 3 weeks after onset of symptoms. Because the largest risk for pertussis-related morbidity and mortality is in infants and young children, it is appropriate to consider antibiotic therapy for pregnant women (or those to be in close contact with the newborn) for up to 6 weeks after onset of cough symptoms. It is also reasonable to consider treatment of those with asthma, chronic obstructive pulmonary disease, age older than 65 years, and/or immunocompromised states.[7] Macrolides, such as a standard 5-day course of azithromycin, are the preferred treatment regimen. Vaccination is an important and effective element in the prevention of this disease.

Additionally, medications, specifically angiotensin-converting enzyme (ACE) inhibitors, may cause a subacute or chronic, nonproductive cough (in up to 15% of patients treated with ACE inhibitors).[8] It is believed that the accumulation of bradykinin, which is typically catalyzed by ACE, may stimulate cough receptors. Generally, cough related to ACE inhibitors begins within 1 week of initiating therapy (although it can be delayed up to 6 months) and resolves within 1 week of discontinuation (although it may last up to 4 weeks).[9] This adverse effect is more common in women and those of Chinese origin.[10] Asthma does not seem to play a role. Cough returns on rechallenge with any ACE inhibitor. If the medication is still indicated, switching to angiotensin receptor antagonists, such as losartan, or other antihypertensives is advised.

Most commonly, chronic cough is caused by upper airway cough syndrome (UACS; secondary to postnasal drip), gastroesophageal reflux, or asthma.[11] UACS and gastroesophageal reflux may also present with subacute cough, although cough of a subacute duration is most often caused by postinfectious etiologies. Its pathogenesis is not entirely understood, but it is thought to be caused by airway inflammation and hyperresponsiveness, mucus hypersecretion, along with impaired clearance.[5]

UACS is the preferred name when referring to cough secondary to postnasal drip. The mechanism of cough is not entirely clear, although it is suspected to be secondary to stimulation of laryngeal cough receptors.[6] The underlying causes include rhinitis (allergic, perennial nonallergic, and vasomotor), acute nasopharyngitis ("the common cold"), and sinusitis. Patients may complain of rhinorrhea, frequent throat clearing, a sensation of dripping or tickle in the back of the throat, or no symptoms at all. Visualization of secretions in the posterior nasopharynx or cobblestoning of the mucosa is suggestive. Because the history and physical examination in UACS may be elusive, empiric treatment may be the only way to confirm the diagnosis.

Asthma-related cough is generally accompanied by wheezing and dyspnea, although cough may be the only symptom in cough-variant asthma. Cough-variant asthma may eventually progress to include wheezing and dyspnea. Factors suggestive of asthma include family history of asthma; personal or family history of atopy; and worsening of cough symptoms on exposure to fumes, fragrances, dust, mold, and cold air. Cough secondary to asthma may also be seasonal or follow an upper respiratory tract infection. As is the case with typical presentations of asthma, spirometry may help reveal obstructive disease. Alternatively, spirometry is normal and bronchoprovocation may be required to demonstrate airway hyperreactivity. However, because the ability for spirometry to discern the cause of chronic cough is poor,[9] the best way to confirm the diagnosis of cough-variant asthma is to observe improvement in symptoms with appropriate asthma therapy.

Gastroesophageal reflux is another frequent cause for prolonged cough. Patients frequently report heartburn or a sour taste in the mouth, although these symptoms may be absent in 40% of patients whose cough is attributable to reflux.[12] Often, cough is worse when the patient is in the recumbent position because it allows for easier reflux from the stomach.[1] Although gastroesophageal reflux is thought to be related to dysfunction of the lower esophageal sphincter, laryngopharyngeal reflux (LPR) is attributed to upper esophageal sphincter dysfunction. Few patients with LPR endorse heartburn. Instead, dysphonia, hoarseness, nonproductive throat clearing, and cough are the hallmark symptoms. Laryngoscopic examination may assist in diagnosing LPR. Hoarseness in patients with significant smoking history, especially in the absence of other signs or symptoms to suggest reflux, should prompt consideration for malignancy.

Lung cancer, a feared diagnosis, is the cause in less than 2% of chronic coughs.[8,13] Lung cancers presenting as cough are often found in the larger, central airways. The physical examination may include wheezes or focal decreased breath sounds, which could suggest tumoral obstruction of the airway. Consider lung cancer in smokers who have a new cough, a change in their usual "smoker's cough," or cough persisting for more than 1 month after smoking cessation.[14] Survival is better in patients ultimately diagnosed with lung cancer whose initial presenting symptom is cough alone, as compared with other presentations.[5]

Chronic bronchitis is defined as cough and sputum production on most days over a 3 month period for 2 or more consecutive years (without any other cause of cough identified). It is almost universally a disease of smokers. Those with airway inflammation caused by exposure to dusts or fumes comprise the small fraction of nonsmokers with chronic bronchitis. Chronic bronchitis is a common condition, because of to the prevalence of cigarette smoking. However, most smokers to do not seek medical care for their cough. Sputum produced in chronic bronchitis is generally clear or white; purulent appearance (or a change in the typical appearance) often signifies respiratory infection and should be treated as such.

Recurrent airway infections and/or inflammation can lead to the development of bronchiectasis. Bronchiectasis is a cyclical condition of airway inflammation and bronchial destruction causing dilation of airways and subsequent impaired mucus clearance and secretion pooling, which in turn worsens inflammation and predisposes for infection. Cough in bronchiectasis is most often productive of copious mucopurulent sputum (which may become frankly purulent and fetid at the time of exacerbation).[15] Although examination may be normal, more frequently adventitial sounds and digital clubbing are usually identified.[16]

Bronchiectasis may affect the lungs diffusely or in specific regions. Regional bronchiectasis is often caused by a prior severe lower respiratory tract infection, whereas multifocal bronchiectasis is often secondary to chronic infection with *Mycobacterium avium* complex, commonly seen in women middle aged and older. In a younger person, consider congenital conditions, such as cystic fibrosis or immunoglobulin deficiency.[6]

Foreign bodies can also lead to a persistent cough. Although more common in children, central nervous system impairment, traumatic endotracheal intubation, and dental procedures predispose adults to aspiration of a foreign body. This should be considered in patients with chronic cough and/or recurrent pneumonia.[17] Foreign bodies may not only be limited to the tracheobronchial tree. Impaction of the auditory canal with a foreign body or cerumen may cause chronic cough via stimulation of the auricular branch of the vagus nerve (otorespiratory reflex).[18]

Tracheobronchomalacia (TBM) is becoming an increasingly recognized cause of respiratory symptoms, including chronic cough. TBM is a condition of excessive dynamic airway collapse, defined by a 50% reduction in cross-sectional area of the central airways. In most adults, the cause of TBM is not known, although it is often seen with other pulmonary conditions. The cough is often of a barking quality; stridor may also be present.[19] Dynamic (inspiratory and expiratory phase) noncontrast chest computed tomography (CT) is the least invasive manner to diagnose TBM, although bronchoscopy may be required.[20]

Other uncommon causes of a chronic cough include arteriovenous malformations, retrotracheal masses, premature ventricular contractions, and psychogenic causes ("tic cough"). The more common previously mentioned diagnoses should be thoroughly ruled out before considering these.

EVALUATION

The initial evaluation for the patient with chronic cough is reliant on a thorough history and physical examination. Important historical aspects include smoking status, current medications, and concurrent symptoms. Eliciting any concerning or systemic symptoms, such as hemoptysis, weight loss, or shortness of breath, should result in a more urgent assessment, which would likely include further diagnostic testing. Additionally, the timing and aggravating and relieving activities can help to localize the potential cause of the cough.

Patients who have had chronic cough warrant a chest radiograph whether they are smokers or not. It is important to recognize that the resolution of routine chest films may not be enough to identify patients with chronic interstitial lung disease or disorders of the airways and mediastinum.[21] In these cases, and in the cases of patients in whom other chronic lung disease is suspected or in patients with warning symptoms, such as hemoptysis or concomitant weight loss, a noncontrast CT scan of the chest should be considered.

When the history and physical examination are suggestive of one of the more common causes of cough, treatment should be initiated accordingly. However, there are data to suggest that even without evidence of a likely cause, an empiric therapeutic trial of targeted medications may be a more efficient and cost-effective strategy in the evaluation of chronic cough.[22,23] With this in mind, one would best approach the patient with cough in a step-wise fashion. First and foremost, all active smokers should be encouraged to stop smoking with the expectation of resolution of cough within several weeks. Any patient on treatment with an ACE inhibitor should have the medication discontinued and symptoms monitored for a few weeks.

Suspected Cause

If the history and physical examination are suggestive of UACS, treatment with an antihistamine or decongestant is favored.[24] In cases where there is a significant component of allergic rhinitis, an intranasal corticosteroid is tried. Treatment duration should last at least 2 weeks but can be extended. If there is a partial response to treatment and UACS is strongly suspected, CT of the sinuses and ENT referral is helpful.

Alternatively, if the leading diagnosis is asthma, pulmonary function testing with spirometry should be performed and the patient should begin a 2- to 4-week trial of a combination inhaled corticosteroid-long acting beta agonist.[25] If there is only minimal improvement with this inhaled regimen, a course of oral steroids is considered.

When LPR or gastroesophageal reflux disease is the cause of cough, treatment should consist of once-daily proton pump inhibitor for at least 8 weeks.[26] Further diagnostic testing for reflux disease is controversial, but in the evaluation of cough, laryngoscopy may be helpful in providing evidence of LPR.

Unidentified Cause

When the history, physical examination, and chest radiograph do not identify a likely cause of chronic cough, an empiric strategy of treatment is suggested.[27] The strategy starts with treatment of UACS as discussed previously. If no improvement, one would investigate for asthma with spirometry and perhaps methacholine challenge and treat empirically. Finally, the patient should undergo a therapeutic trial for reflux.

If symptoms persist at this point, further diagnostic testing should be considered including a CT scan of the chest (if not previously ordered) and referral to a specialist for invasive procedures. These might include a referral to otolaryngology for laryngoscopy, gastroenterology for pH probe monitoring, or pulmonary medicine for inspection bronchoscopy.

When no cause is identified, treating symptomatically for cough hypersensitivity syndrome with neurologic medications, such as gabapentin, has been shown to improve quality of life in patients with persistent chronic cough.[28,29]

SUMMARY

Cough is one of the most common presenting symptoms in the primary care setting and has a significant impact of a patient's quality of life.[30] A targeted approach to the assessment and treatment of cough involves identifying concerning signs and symptoms, tailoring therapies for identified etiologies of cough, and initiating an empiric and staged trial of therapy toward the most common causes in situations where no plausible diagnosis is established. Careful consideration must be paid to the potential for multiple concomitant causes of cough and, occasionally, treatment for two or more of the more common causes may be needed in coordination to eliminate the symptom completely.

CLINICS CARE POINTS

- Cough is one of the most common presenting symptoms in the outpatient setting and is classified by its duration.
- Etiologies of cough vary depending on the duration of the symptoms and are often identified by a complete history.
- While acute and subacute cough are mostly often related to an infectious in etiology, chronic cough is most commonly related to post nasal drip, asthma or gastroesophageal reflux disease.
- The evaluation of chronic cough is influenced by smoking status, current medications and concurrent symptoms.
- If there is a suspected cause of chronic cough, empiric treatment for this etiology is cost-effective and can prove therapeutic.
- When there is uncertain etiology of chronic cough, further evaluation with imaging modalities, such as CT scan, laryngoscopy, bronchoscopy or pH probe monitoring may be indicated.

DISCLOSURES

The authors have nothing to disclose.

REFERENCES

1. Sharma S, Hashmi MF, Alhajjaj MS. Cough. [Updated 2020 Feb 14]. In: StatPearls [Internet]. Treasure Island (FL): StatPearls Publishing; 2020. Available at: https://www.ncbi.nlm.nih.gov/books/NBK493221/.

2. Irwin RS, Curley FJ, French CL. Chronic cough. The spectrum and frequency of causes, key components of the diagnostic evaluation, and outcome of specific therapy. Am Rev Respir Dis 1990;141:640–7.
3. Ekici A, Llesi S, Aslan H, et al. Troublesome cough as the sole manifestation of pulmonary embolism. Respir Med Case Rep 2019;28:100861.
4. Canning B, Chang AB, Bolser DC, et al. Anatomy and neurophysiology of cough. Chest 2014;146(6):1633–44.
5. Braman S. Postinfectious cough. Chest 2006;129(1):138S–46S.
6. De Serres G, Shadmani R, Duval B, et al. Morbidity of pertussis in adolescents and adults. J Infect Dis 2000;182(1):174.
7. Mbayei SA, Faulkner A, Miner C, et al. Severe pertussis infections in the United States, 2011-2015. Clin Infect Dis 2019;69(2):218.
8. Israili ZH, Hall WD. Cough and angioneurotic edema associated with angiotensin converting enzyme inhibitor therapy. A review of the literature and pathophysioloyg. Ann Intern Med 1992;117(3):234.
9. Irwin RS, Curley FJ, French CL, et al. Chronic cough. Am Rev Respir Dis 1990; 141(3):640–7.
10. Tseng DS, Kwong J, Rezvani F, et al. Angiotensin-converting enzyme-related cough among Chinese-Americans. Am J Med 2010;123(2):183.
11. Irwin RS, Baumann MH, Bolser DC, et al. Diagnosis and management of cough executive summary: ACCP evidence-based clinical practice guidelines. Chest 2006;129(1 Suppl):1S–23S.
12. Irwin RS, Zawacki JK, Curley FJ, et al. Chronic cough as the sole presenting manifestation of gastroesophageal reflux. Am Rev Respir Dis 1989;140(5):1294.
13. Hyde L, Hyde CI. Clinical manifestations of lung cancer. Chest 1974;65(3): 299–306.
14. Athey VL, Walters SJ, Rogers TK. Symptoms at lung cancer diagnosis are associated with major differences in prognosis. Thorax 2018;73(12):1177.
15. Smyrnios NA, Irwin RS, Curley FJ. Chronic cough with a history of excessive sputum production. The spectrum and frequency of causes, key components of the diagnostic evaluation and outcome of specific therapy. Chest 1995;108(4):991.
16. Bates D, Macklem P, Christie R. Respiratory function in disease. 2nd edition. Philadelphia: W. B. Saunders; 1971. p. 231.
17. Kam JC, Doraiswamy V, Dieguez JF, et al. Foreign body aspiration presenting with asthma-like symptoms. Case Rep Med 2013;2013:317104. Article ID 317104.
18. Feldman JI, Woodworth WF. "Cause for intractable chronic cough: Arnold's nerve. Arch Otolaryngol Head Neck Surg 1993;119(9):1042.
19. Choi S, Lawlor C, Rahbar R, et al. Diagnosis, classification, and management of pediatric tracheo-bronchomalacia: a review. JAMA Otolaryngol Head Neck Surg 2019;145(3):265–75.
20. Buitrago D, Wilson JL, Pasikh M, et al. Current concepts in severe adult tracheobronchomalacia: evaluation and treatment. J Thorac Dis 2017;9(1):E57–66.
21. Brown KK. Chronic cough due to chronic pulmonary interstitial diseases. ACCP evidence-based practice guidelines. Chest 2006;129:180S–5S.
22. Lin L, Poh KL, Tim TK. Empirical treatment of chronic cough: a cost-effectiveness analysis. Proc AMIA Symp. 2001;383–7.
23. Pratter MR, Bartter T, Akers S, et al. An algorithmic approach to chronic cough. Ann Intern Med 1993;119:977–83.
24. Pratter MR. Chronic upper airway cough syndrome secondary to rhinosinus diseases. ACCP evidence-based clinical practice guidelines. Chest 2006;129:59S–62S.

25. Global Initiative for Asthma. Global Strategy for Asthma Management and Prevention 2020. Available at: www.ginasthma.org.

26. Katz P, Gerson LB, Vera MF, et al. Guidelines for the diagnosis and management of gastroesophageal reflux disease. Am J Gastroenterol 2013;108:308–28.

27. Yu Li, Xu X, Hang J, et al. Efficacy of sequential three-step empirical therapy for chronic cough. Ther Adv Respir Dis 2017;11(6):225–32.

28. Ryan NM, Birring SS, Gibson PG. Gabapentin for refractory chronic cough: a randomized, double-blind, placebo-controlled trial. Lancet 2012;380(9853):1583–9.

29. Gibson P, Wang G, McGarvey L, et al. Treatment of unexplained chronic cough: CHEST guideline and expert panel report. Chest 2016;149(1):27–44.

30. Young EC, Smith JA. Quality of life in patients with chronic cough. Ther Adv Respir Dis 2010;4(1):49–55.

Headaches in Adults in Primary Care
Evaluation, Diagnosis, and Treatment

Melissa McNeil, MD, MPH, MACP*

KEYWORDS

- Headache • Tension-type headache • Migraine headache • Abortive therapy
- Preventive therapy

KEY POINTS

- Headaches are traditionally classified as primary (tension-type headaches, migraines, cluster headaches) or secondary headaches (intracranial pathology, vascular disease, medication overuse headaches).
- Headaches can be diagnosed with a careful history and physical with attention to red flag symptoms.
- Treating migraine headaches has 2 components: treating the acute headache (abortive therapy) and preventing the onset of later headaches (prophylactic therapy).
- Early treatment of acute symptoms is important with careful attention to avoiding over-treatment to prevent overuse headaches.
- Prophylactic therapy for for either Tension-type headaches or migraine headaches is indicated if the headaches are frequent, long lasting, or are associated with significant functional impairment.

INTRODUCTION

Headache is one of the most common symptom presentations in primary care[1] with more than 90% of all primary headaches falling into 2 categories, tension-type headache and migraine headache.[2] It is estimated that more than 3 billion individuals worldwide suffer from headaches, with 1.89 billion patients with tension-type headaches and 1.04 billion with migraine headaches. Although tension headaches are more common in the population than migraine headaches, migraine is the most frequent etiology of headaches in patients seeking treatment because of the increased disability of migraine headaches. Migraine headaches are the second most disabling medical condition worldwide, impacting all domains of life. Given the prevalence of headaches in the population and frequency with which patients with headaches present in primary care settings, an understanding of the different headache syndromes and their management should be a part of every primary care physician's repertoire.

University of Pittsburg, Pittsburgh, PA, USA
* UPMC Montefiore Hospital, 200 Lothrop St, Suite 9W, Pittsburgh, PA 15213.
E-mail address: mcneilma@upmc.edu

Med Clin N Am 105 (2021) 39–53
https://doi.org/10.1016/j.mcna.2020.09.005
0025-7125/21/© 2020 Elsevier Inc. All rights reserved.

This review focuses on the 2 most common headache syndromes encountered in primary care practice—tension-type headache and migraine headaches.

CLASSIFICATION OF HEADACHES

Headaches are traditionally classified as primary (tension-type headaches, migraines, cluster headaches) or secondary headaches (intracranial pathology, vascular disease, medication overuse headaches) and can be diagnosed with a careful history and physical examination with attention to red flag symptoms. Important historical features include location, characteristics of the headache, degree of functional impairment, duration, and associated symptoms. The physical examination should focus on discriminators of secondary etiologies: vital signs (blood pressure and pulse), bruits of the head and neck, palpation of the temporal arteries, and palpation of the head, neck, and shoulder muscles, with a detailed neurologic examination, including cranial nerve testing, funduscopy, and symmetry of motor, reflex, cerebellar, and sensory testing. Patient characteristics with low risk for secondary disease include: age 50 years or younger, features typical of a primary headache syndrome, history of similar headache with no change in usual pattern, and a normal physical examination (**Table 1**). Patients who meet these criteria and have no red flag symptom do not require imaging. Red flag symptoms include[3] onset after age 50; pattern change (eg, worst headache of your life); positional headache or headache precipitated by sneezing, coughing, or exercise; symptoms such as fever or history of neoplasm or trauma; and papilledema or neurologic deficit. The presence of any red flag symptoms should trigger further evaluation including brain imaging (**Table 2**).

TENSION-TYPE HEADACHE
Pathophysiology and Headache Characteristics

Tension-type headache is the most common headache in the general population and the second-most prevalent disorder in the world[4] (**Table 3**). Tension-type headache presents as an undifferentiated headache syndrome that is characterized by a bilateral headache of mild to moderate intensity that is nonthrobbing and has no associated symptoms such as sensitivity to light or sound or nausea or vomiting. The pain is described as pressure or bandlike. The pain is not aggravated by routine physical activity, such as walking or climbing stairs. The physical examination may demonstrate increased pericranial muscle tenderness of the head, neck, or shoulders. The diagnosis is clinical and neuroimaging is not required in the absence of red flag findings, as discussed elsewhere in this article. The headache can last days and patients can usually function through their headaches.

There are 3 main subtypes recognized by the International Headache Classification:

- Infrequent episodic tension-type headache: headache less than 1 day per month (63.5% of tension-type headache patients)
- Frequent episodic tension-type headache: headache 1 to 14 days per month (21.6% of tension-type headache patients)
- Chronic episodic tension-type headache: headache 15 or more days per month (0.9% of tension-type headache patients)

A population-based study in the United States found that the prevalence of episodic tension-type headache peaked in the fourth decade with a decreasing prevalence with advancing age.[5] Women and whites have a slightly higher prevalence of tension-type headache than men and black patients. The societal impact is high for patients with

Table 1
Characteristic of common primary headache syndromes

Characteristic	Tension Type	Migraine	Headache
Demographics	Slightly more common in women; 1 year prevalence for episodic tension-type headache 38.3%, chronic tension-type headache 2.2%; higher prevalence in white patients		
Patient appearance	Variable; generally patient remains active and functional or may retreat	Uncomfortable; prefers dark and quiet room; function is impaired	Generally remains functional
Location	Unilateral in 70%; bilateral or global in 30%;	Bilateral, usually temporal but rarely generalizes to the entire head	Always unilateral; classically begins in the eye or around the temple
Duration	4–72 h; may be evident all day (present upon awakening and there when going to sleep)	30 min to 7 d	15 min to 3 h
Characteristics	Mild to moderate intensity; bilateral; nonthrobbing	Pressure; tightness; often described as band-like	Acute onset—reaches maximum intensity within minutes; pain is severe and incapacitating
Associated symptoms	None	May have associated aura (visual or other neurologic deficit); Nausea and/or vomiting; Photophobia or phonophobia;	Tearing and eye redness on the same side as the headache; rhinorrhea; seating; Horner syndrome; sensitivity to alcohol

Table 2
Red flag symptoms requiring further evaluation

Symptom	Example
Age	After 50
Pattern change	Worst headache of your life
Positional headache	Exacerbated with change
Precipitating factors	Sneezing, coughing, exercise
High risk history	Fever, neoplasm, trauma
Physical examination findings	Papilledema, neurologic deficit

episodic tension-type headache reporting an average of 9 lost work days and 5 reduced effectiveness days per year.[5]

The pathophysiology of tension-type headache is unclear, but probably multifactorial. Current models propose that activation of myofascial pain receptors is the underlying cause of episodic tension-type headache, whereas sensitization of pain pathways in the central nervous system owing to prolonged stimuli from pericranial myofascial tissues is responsible for the conversion from episodic to chronic tension-type headache. Studies of pain tolerance in these patients have suggested generalized hyperalgesia in patients with chronic tension-type headache. Thus, increased sensitivity to pain in both the central and the peripheral nervous systems is thought to play a critical role in the pathogenesis of tension-type headache.[6] Spasm of the pericranial muscles was long thought to be important in the pathophysiology of tension-type headache, but this construct is no longer considered a factor. There are minimal if any genetic predispositions to tension-type headache.

Treatment of Acute Tension-Type Headache

Most patients with tension-type headache self-treat using over-the-counter medications without consulting a medical provider. When managing tension-type headache, several principles (albeit not evidence based) are thought to guide therapy.

Table 3
Recommended pharmacologic treatment of tension-type headaches

Medication	Dose	Caveats
Acute treatment		
Pain medications		
Acetaminophen	1000 mg	Enhanced with caffeine
Ibuprofen	400 mg	
Ketoprofen	25 mg	
Aspirin	1000 mg	Enhanced with caffeine
Chronic treatment		
Antidepressants		
Amitriptyline	10–25 mg	Many side effects
Anticonvulsants		
Topiramate	25–00 mg	Reduction at 3 mo

- Because abortive therapy is more effective for migraine headache when given early, it is generally presumed to be more effective for tension-type headache when given as soon as possible after headache onset, although no evidence is available to support that belief.
- Similarly, recommendations are to start with a maximum initial medication dose with the hope of eliminating later doses; the effectiveness of analgesics decreases with increasing headache duration and frequency.
- Chronic tension-type headache is often associated with stress, anxiety, and depression,[7] and analgesics are usually of limited benefit in this setting.
- Avoiding medication overuse headache is a crucial goal of therapy and requires extensive patient education and counseling. The recommendations are that over-the-counter combination medications should be limited to 9 treatment days per month and nonsteroidal anti-inflammatory drugs (NSAIDs) should be limited to 15 or fewer days per month.
- Opioids and butalbital containing analgesics should be avoided owing to their high potential for misuse, including inducing medication overuse headaches.

Clinical trial evidence supports using simple analgesic agents like acetaminophen, aspirin, and NSAIDs as initial therapy.[8] A systematic review of randomized controlled trials concluded that acetaminophen 1000 mg, ibuprofen 400 mg, and ketoprofen 25 mg were more effective than placebo for achieving a pain-free state at 2 hours. Aspirin (1000 mg) was less effective but better than placebo with its effectiveness modest at best with pain-free rates at 2 hours ranging from 16% to 37%. Overall, NSAIDs are preferred because they are less likely to lead to medication overuse headaches than acetaminophen. The role of combination agents is also unclear. Several studies have suggested that adding caffeine to either aspirin or acetaminophen was superior to either agent alone.

Prevention of Tension-Type Headaches

Prophylactic therapy for tension-type headache is indicated if the headaches are frequent, long lasting, or are associated with significant functional impairment. Generally, a frequency of more than 10 headache days per month warrants preventive treatment. Evidence for pharmacologic therapy is limited, but a recent review[9] suggested that the evidence is most robust for tricyclic antidepressants. Other suggested medications include mirtazapine, venlafaxine, topiramate, and gabapentin and the muscle relaxant tizanidine.

Antidepressants

A 2017 meta-analysis[10] supported the contention that tricyclics are therapeutic for tension-type headache prevention. Headache frequency was reduced by 4.8 headaches per month in patients with very frequent headaches (21 headaches per month) and analgesic use was decreased. However, given the headache frequency, this effect was modest at best. Recommendations for starting tricyclic therapy include starting at the lowest dose (10 mg of amitriptyline) and waiting at least 2 weeks before increasing the dose. A maximum dose of 100 to 125 mg of amitriptyline is recommended. Benefits may continue to be seen for up to 3 months after initiating therapy. Nortriptyline and protriptyline are alternatives if amitriptyline is poorly tolerated. Side effects limit the usefulness of this medication and include dry mouth, constipation, palpitations, orthostatic hypotension, weight gain, blurry vision, and urinary retention. Confusion is also common in the elderly. In addition, these medications are associated with an increased risk of cardiac conduction abnormalities and preexisting conduction system disease precludes their use. There are less robust data supporting the use of mirtazapine and venlafaxine; in contrast, evidence suggests that selective serotonin reuptake inhibitors are only effective for the treatment of tension-type headache in patients with depression.[11]

Anticonvulsants
There is 1 open-label study of 51 patients with tension-type headache treated with topiramate (starting at 25 mg/d increasing to 100 mg/d), which reported a decrease in headache frequency after 3 months.[12] The medication is generally well-tolerated, but there are many side effects that include paresthesia, anorexia, weight loss, fatigue, difficulty with memory and concentration, nausea, and alterations in taste. Side effects are more common at higher doses and 30% of patients on 200 mg/d had to have the drug withdrawn. It is also a teratogenic, so birth control is critical in women of reproductive age. There is very little evidence to support the use of gabapentin for the treatment of tension-type headache. The 1 study that evaluated the use of gabapentin in tension-type headache prevention was limited by the fact that 58 of the 95 patients studied had a combination of migraine and tension-type headache. High-dose gabapentin (2400 mg) was associated with a significant decrease in headache-free days, but it is unclear if the benefit was due to migraine reduction.[13]

Other pharmacologic interventions
The muscle relaxant tizanidine has been evaluated in several small studies with conflicting results. Trigger point injections with lidocaine may be promising; several small trials suggest a reduction in headache frequency and acute medication use[14] but the studies are small and more data is needed. There is little data to support the use of botulinum toxin injections. A 2012 meta-analysis evaluated onabotulinumtoxin A (botulinum toxin type A) as a preventive treatment for tension-type headache and found no statistically significant decrease in headache frequency.[15]

Behavioral therapies
Given the lack of benefit of pharmacologic interventions in the prevention of tension-type headache, behavioral treatments should be a part of every headache prevention strategy despite limited data showing efficacy. Recommended behavioral modifications include the following: regulation of sleep, exercise, and meals; cognitive-behavioral therapy; relaxation techniques; biofeedback; and stress management.[16] Studies suggest that stress and mental tension are the most frequently identified triggers for tension-type headache and developing coping skills is an important part of any behavioral therapy. The analysis of the effectiveness of behavioral interventions is limited with small studies, many of which lack of methodologic rigor. The most robust data is for biofeedback. A 2008 meta-analysis concluded that biofeedback was more effective than headache monitoring alone, and that this benefit was increased by adding relaxation therapy.[17] A combination of stress management therapy and tricyclic medication has been shown to be more effective than either therapy alone.[18] There are limited studies that support both Tai Chi[19] and yoga.[20] One randomized controlled trial of 15 weeks of Tai Chi in 47 patients with tension-type headache found a reduction in both headache impact and an increase in quality of life. There is 1 randomized controlled trial that suggests that yoga may be beneficial, but the numbers are small. It is unclear whether headache frequency and/or intensity improved or if overall coping and overall perception of wellness was enhanced.

Other therapies
Both acupuncture and physical therapies (including exercises, traction, spinal manipulation, transcutaneous electoral nerve stimulation, electromagnetic therapy, and

ultrasound therapy) have all been proposed. Several meta-analyses have tried to look at the benefit of such therapies,[21] but the trials are small and have methodologic problems. Results are heterogeneous with inconsistent benefit reported. Although there is a lack of clear benefit in well-done studies, these treatments are low risk and may offer a decrease in some patients and should be considered as alternative therapies.

MIGRAINE HEADACHE
Pathophysiology and Headache Characteristics

The traditional understanding that the pathophysiology of migraine headache is secondary to vasodilation and that the aura of migraine is cause by vasoconstriction is no longer considered accurate[22] (**Table 4**). The current understanding underlying migraine suggests that the primary insult is a neuronal aberration that leads to a

Table 4 Recommended pharmacologic treatment of migraine headaches		
Medication	**Dose**	**Caveats**
Acute treatment		
Pain medications		
Acetaminophen	1000 mg	Do not underdose!
Ibuprofen	400–600 mg	
Naproxen	275–825 mg	
Diclofenac	50–100 mg	
Aspirin	1000 mg	
Triptans		
Sumatriptan	50–100 mg	Oral, nasal, SQ injection
Rizatriptan	10 mg	Oral only
Eletriptan	80 mg	Oral only
Almotriptan	12.5 mg	Oral only
Antiemetics		
Metoclopramide	10 mg PO or IV	Give with antihistamine
Prochlorperazine	10 mg IV	Give with antihistamine
Chronic treatment		
Beta-blockers		
Metoprolol	5 mg BID to 200 mg/d	
Propranolol	40 mg BID to 160 QD	
Timolol	5 mg QD to 30 mg/d	Higher doses BID
Antidepressants		
Amitriptyline	10 mg up to 50 mg	Titrate every 2–4 wk
Venlafaxine	25 up to 150 mg	
Anticonvulsants		
Topiramate	25 mg to 200 mg BID	Teratogenic
Valproic acid	500–1500 mg	Teratogenic
Calcitonin gene-related peptide antagonist		
Erenumab	70–140 mg q month	Last resort

Abbreviations: BID, 2 times per day; IM, intramuscularly; IV, intravenously; PO, by mouth; SQ, subcutaneously; QD, daily.

spreading of self-propagating depolarization that spreads across the cortex.[23] This spreading depolarization is thought to both cause the aura and to activate the trigeminovascular system, which then leads to inflammatory changes in the pain receptors of the meninges, subsequently leading to the pain of migraine headache. Vasoactive peptides are released in response to the neurogenic inflammation, which in turn then cause vasodilation and plasma protein extravasation. When vasodilation occurs it is thus thought to be a secondary phenomenon. Although the use of serotonin-augmenting agents is the mainstay in the treatment of acute migraine headaches, the role of serotonin in the initiation of migraine headaches remains uncertain. There is some evidence that baseline low levels of serotonin may enhance the activation of the trigeminovascular nociceptive pain pathways owing to a deficit in the serotonin-mediated descending pain inhibitory system.[24,25] There is also a complex genetic component underlying the etiology of migraines. The risk of migraine headaches is 3 times greater in relatives of migraineurs than the population at large.[26] No specific Mendelian pattern of inheritance has been identified. It is thought that the familial basis of migraine headaches is due to a different genetic threshold between excitatory and inhibitory channels in the nervous system that makes patients more susceptible to a migraine attack.

Migraine is a recurrent headache disorder that classically has 4 phases[27,28]. (1) Prodrome (prevalence 77%): These symptoms may occur 24–48 hours before the onset of headache and consist of a wide variety of symptoms including depression, euphoria, irritability, and food cravings. (2) Aura (prevalence 25%): A typical migraine aura is characterized by the gradual development of either positive and negative neurologic symptoms lasting no longer than 1 hour and having complete resolution. Positive symptoms are classically visual (bright lines, shapes, objects) or auditory (tinnitus, noises, music) but can also be somatosensory or motor (paresthesia, jerking). Negative symptoms include loss of vision, hearing, feeling, or body movement. Patients may also experience auras without headache, known as a migraine equivalent. Negative symptoms or auras without headache are often confused with transient ischemic attacks. (3) Migraine headache: The details of the headache are the most important diagnostic consideration in approaching a patient with a headache syndrome. Classically, migraine headaches are described as unilateral, throbbing, and moderate to severe in intensity. Associated symptoms include photophobia, phonophobia, and nausea and vomiting. Symptoms increase over a course of 1 to 2 hours and can last 4 hours to several days. Commonly attacks with resolve with sleep. (4) Postdrome: After resolution there may be a postdromal phase characterized by pain owing to sudden head movement in the area of the previous headache. Patients may feel either exhausted or have euphoria.

A careful history and physical examination is the most important diagnostic tool for the diagnosis of migraine headaches. Careful attention to the timing, location, nature, and associated features of the headache is critical. The neurologic examination should be nonfocal. Yet, despite clear guidelines, many migraine headaches are misdiagnosed. For example, a significant number of migraine headaches are accompanied by nasal congestion and are misdiagnosed as sinus headaches.[26] Given the challenges in diagnosis, a number of diagnostic questionnaires have been developed and validated. The easiest to remember is the ID Migraine.[29] Patients with 2 or more headaches in the previous 3 months were asked the following: (1) *Photophobia*: Did light bother you? (2) *Incapacity*: Did your headaches limit your ability to work, study, or do what you needed to do for at least 1 day? (3) *Nausea*: Did you feel nauseated or sick to your stomach? This diagnostic screen is considered positive if 2 of the questions are answered yes. In a systematic review of more than 500 studies the pooled sensitivity of this 3-question tool was 0.84 and the pooled specificity was 0.76.[30] The mnemonic PIN (Pain, Incapacity, Nausea) is an easy way to remember the questions used in this screen. Another commonly used screening tool is the POUND mnemonic asking 5 yes or no questions: pulsatile, onset 4 to 72 hours, unilateral, nausea/vomiting, and disabling. If 3 questions are answered yes, the likelihood ratio for a migraine is 3.5; if 4 questions are answered yes, the likelihood ratio is 24. Interestingly adding associated symptoms of photophobia/phonophobia did not enhance performance criteria.[31] An even easier screen is asking if the headache was disabling. In 1 study, this simple question identified migraine in 136 or 146 patients (93%) with episodic migraine headaches.[32]

Treatment of Acute Migraine Headache

Treating migraine headaches has 2 components: treating the acute headache (abortive therapy) and preventing the onset of later headaches (prophylactic therapy). This section reviews commonly used measures for the acute treatment of migraine. Several observations guide therapeutic recommendations: (1) abortive therapies are more effective the earlier they are administered in the course of the headache, (2) a single large dose of a medication is more effective than repeated smaller doses of medications, and (3) many oral medications are of limited effectiveness because migraine induces gastric stasis, which leads to poor absorption. Treatment options consist primarily of simple analgesics, migraine-specific agents, and antiemetics.

Simple analgesics
Both acetaminophen and NSAIDs including aspirin have been show to be efficacious. A randomized, placebo-based trial of acetaminophen at a dose of 1000 mg in patients with self-reported migraines demonstrated relief in both pain and functional disability.[33] Many NSAIDs have reported efficacy in acute migraine treatment and include aspirin (900–1000 mg), ibuprofen (400–600 mg), naproxen (275–825 mg), and diclofenac (50–100 mg) among others. This suggests that all NSAIDs may be effective in treating migraine patients both with and without aura if appropriately high doses are used. One of the most common mistakes is the underdosing the initial dose of NSAIDs. Head-to-head comparisons are limited, so if 1 medication does not work then another medication should be tried. Remember also that acetaminophen can be used in combination with NSAIDs. The over-the-counter combination of acetaminophen, aspirin, and caffeine has also been shown to be effective.[34] Parenteral ketorolac (30 mg intravenously [IV] or 60 mg intramuscularly [IM]) can be considered in patient with significant nausea or vomiting.

Triptans
Triptans are 1 b/1d serotonin agonists and are effective migraine-specific treatments to stop acute migraine headaches.[35] Two available preparations have both oral and nonoral administrations: sumatriptan (oral, nasal spray, or subcutaneous injection) and zolmitriptan (oral and nasal). The remaining agents include naratriptan, rizatriptan, almotriptan, eletriptan, and frovatriptan and are only available for oral use. There is a paucity of trials comparing the triptans head to head, so the choice of an initial agent may be influenced by availability and desired route of administration. A meta-analysis of the oral agents suggested that the most effective agents were rizatriptan (10 mg dose), eletriptan (80 mg dose), and almotriptan (12.5 mg dose).[36] Naratriptan and frovatriptan were found to be slower in onset and less efficacious overall. Dosing is important and these medications are often underdosed. For example, oral sumatriptan is given at a starting dose of 50 to 100 mg, which may be repeated once after 2 hours

(maximum dose in 24 hours is 200 mg). The 100-mg dose of sumatriptan is more effective but has more side effects. Subcutaneous sumatriptan dosing (6 mg) has a more rapid onset and is more effective than oral sumatriptan, but has more adverse effects including injection site reactions, chest heaviness, flushing, dizziness, and paresthesia. Because head-to-head trials are lacking, the choice of triptan can be individualized; delivery routes may help to guide the decision making. Early administration of the medication and adequate dosing are the factors most likely to predict success. Concern has been raised about triptan use and subsequent cardiovascular events, but a systematic review of observational studies found no association,[37] although these medications were prescribed to lower risk patients. It is also recommended that triptans not be prescribed in patients with hemiplegic migraines, basilar migraines, a history of ischemic strokes or myocardial infarction, angina, uncontrolled hypertension, or pregnancy.[38] A final important note is that, although the combination of a triptan with a serotonin reuptake inhibitor has raised concerns about the possibility of precipitating serotonin syndrome, this risk is so low to nonexistent[39] that most headache experts recommend using triptans in combination with serotonin reuptake inhibitors when indicated.

Antiemetics
Metoclopramide (IV), chlorpromazine (IM), and prochlorperazine (IM) can all be used both as monotherapy for acute migraine headaches or as adjunctive therapy with NSAIDs. Metoclopramide seems to be slightly less effective than either of the other agents but is better tolerated with less risk of QT prolongation than the other medications. Intravenous diphenhydramine (12.5–25.0 mg every hour for 2 hours) is commonly given with these medications to prevent the acute dystonic reactions, which are common and distressing with these medications. In contrast to IV or IM preparations, oral antiemetics are less likely to be effective. Ondansetron for use in acute migraine treatment is less studied, and has a high incidence of headache as a side effect.

Other agents
Less commonly used agents that are poorly defined in their place in the treatment of migraines include lasmiditan (selective serotonin IF receptor agonist), calcitonin-gene related peptide antagonists, and ergotamines. Parenteral treatment with dexamethasone in addition to other abortive therapies has been shown to reduce the rate of early migraine recurrence after initial treatment[40] and may be considered for patients requiring emergency room treatment. Finally, just a reminder that opioids and barbiturates should never be used for the acute treatment of migraines because of limited efficacy, high risk of rebound headaches, and a risk of developing dependence.

Summary
The severity of the attack along with the presence of nausea or vomiting should guide the initial therapy. For milder attacks with no gastrointestinal symptoms, simple analgesics such as acetaminophen or NSAIDs may suffice. They are preferred both because they are cost effective and because they are less likely to cause side effects than the migraine-specific agents. In addition, antiemetics should be considered if there is nausea or vomiting. For moderate attacks with no gastrointestinal symptoms, oral migraine specific agents are first line with or without NSAIDs. The timing and dosage of the initial medications chosen are critical for effective intervention.

Prevention of Migraine Headaches

Prophylactic therapy for migraineurs is recommended for patients with frequent and/ or disabling migraines that do not respond adequately to abortive therapy. More than 4 headaches per month or headaches that last longer than 12 hours are considered indications for preventive therapy.[41] The goals of therapy are to decrease the frequency and severity of the attacks and to improve responsiveness to acute therapy to decrease the associated disability and to help prevent progression to chronic migraines. There are 2 mainstays to preventive therapy. The first is to identify and modify any and all migraine triggers whenever possible; the second is pharmacologic therapy for the prevention of migraines.

In 1 retrospective study, 75% of patients reported at least 1 migraine trigger.[42] Common migraine triggers include emotional stress (80%), estrogen-related changes in women (65%), skipping meals (57%), weather changes (53%), and sleep disturbances (50%). Other common triggers include alcohol (especially wine) and specific foods (especially those including nitrates and aspartame). Asking patients to keep a headache diary to identify individual triggers and then providing counseling and education about trigger factor modification is a critical and often overlooked management strategy for preventing migraines. Avoiding overuse of acute headache therapies such as analgesics and triptans to prevent rebound headaches is also a key component of preventive therapy.

With regard to pharmacologic therapy, 4 classes of drugs have been shown to be effective in the prevention of migraines: beta-blockers, antidepressants, anticonvulsants, and calcitonin gene-related peptide antagonists. General principles of preventive therapy, regardless of the medication chosen, include starting at a low dose increasing gradually until benefit, side effect, or maximum dosage is achieved. Studies have suggested that the benefit of any drug or dosage is unlikely to be noted before 4 weeks and may continue to increase for up to 3 to 6 months for any given medication. Patient education and counseling regarding the extended time needed to assess the benefit of any preventive therapy is critical to avoid patient discontinuation of medications before an effective therapeutic trial has been achieved. Initial treatment should be individualized with attention to comorbid disorders to help with choice of agent; in general, calcitonin gene-related peptide antagonists are not considered to be first-line agents. Approximate 50% to 75% of patients given any of these 3 classes of drugs with have a 50% decrease in headaches.[43]

Beta-blockers

Data from randomized, controlled trials has established the efficacy of metoprolol, propranolol, and timolol for migraine prevention.[44] Lesser evidence suggests but does not establish the efficacy of calcium channel blockers, angiotensin-converting enzyme inhibitors, and angiotensin receptor blockers. Recommended doses for commonly used beta-blockers include the following options: propranolol twice daily starting at a daily dose of 40 mg, with a dose range of 40 to 160 mg/d; metoprolol twice daily starting at a daily dose of 5 mg, with a dose range of 50 to 200 mg/d; and timolol 5 mg starting once daily, with a dose range of 10 to 30 mg/d in 2 divided doses. It can take several weeks for headache improvement to manifest and each dose should be maintained for 3 months before either titrating the medication up or deciding that the medication has failed. There are many comorbid conditions that limit the use of beta-blockers, including bradycardia, hypotension, peripheral vascular disease, depression, and reactive airways disease.

Antidepressants

A 2012 guideline from the American Academy of Neurology concluded that amitriptyline and venlafaxine were effective for migraine prevention.[44] Amitriptyline is started at a dose of 10 mg at bedtime with a titration to a daily dose of up to 50 mg at bedtime. Although nortriptyline, doxepin, and protriptyline are commonly used for migraine prevention, only amitriptyline has data supporting its use. Tricyclic side effects were discussed elsewhere in this article.

Anticonvulsants

Both topiramate and valproate have been established to be more effective for migraine prevention than placebo.[44] Gabapentin has been used, but data are lacking. The starting dose of topiramate is 25 mg/d with a slow titration by 25 mg weekly to a maximum dose of 200 mg twice daily (or the highest tolerated dose). Randomized trials showed that a minimum of 100 mg of topiramate daily was required for symptoms reduction. About 50% of patients demonstrated a 50% decrease in headache frequency. Valproate is also effective at doses ranging from 500 to 1500 mg/d. Higher doses are associated with more side effects that include nausea, lethargy, tremor, dizziness, weight gain, and hair loss. It is also teratogenic, so again birth control is critical.

Calcitonin gene-related peptide antagonists

Erenumab is a human monoclonal antibody that binds to and inhibits the calcitonin gene-related peptide receptor. The medication is modestly effective to prevent migraines; in a study of patients who had failed other medications randomized to 140 mg subcutaneously or placebo, 30% had a 50% or greater decrease in headache days.[45] The starting dose is 70 mg subcutaneously once monthly, which can be increased to 140 mg monthly if needed. The most common side effect is site injection reactions.

Other agents

A host of other agents have been used for migraine prevention. The 2012 American Association of Neurology review[44] concluded that feverfew, magnesium riboflavin, and certain NSAIDS (including ibuprofen and naproxen) may be effective. In addition, several randomized placebo-controlled trials have concluded that botulinum toxic type A injection therapy is effective for the treatment of chronic migraine only ($\geq$15 headache days per month).

SUMMARY

Headaches are common in primary care practices with 90% of primary headaches being either tension-type headache or migraine headache. The diagnosis is made by a careful history and physical with particular attention to the identification of red flag signs and symptoms. Imaging is generally not warranted unless concerning findings are identified. Several general principles underlie the acute treatment of either type of headache with early initiation of therapy and adequate dosing at first dose. Careful attention to avoid too frequent administration of acute therapy is important to minimize medication overuse headaches. Opioids should always be avoided. Preventive treatment is indicated for frequent headaches of either type, but the data are better to support the prevention of migraine headache. Successful treatment requires the initiation of low-dose medication with careful titration and monitoring of headache frequency over months. Finally, behavioral strategies are important in both types of headache and should be a part of any comprehensive headache management plan.

CLINICS CARE POINTS

- Approximately 90% of all primary headache syndromes are tension-type headache or migraine headache; chronic sinus problems, hypertension, and eye strain are commonly diagnosed as causes of headaches. Headaches may worsen with these conditions, but they are rarely the primary cause. Many of these are migraine headaches.
- Both tension-type headache and migraine headache are diagnosed by history and physical diagnosis; in the absence of red flag signs and symptoms, imaging is rarely indicated.
- Abortive therapies for both tension-type headache and migraine headache are more effective the earlier they are administered in the course of the headache and a single large dose of a medication is more effective than repeated smaller doses of medications.
- Avoiding medication overuse headache is a crucial goal of therapy and requires extensive patient education and counseling; episodic treatment medications should be limited to 9 treatment days per month with NSAIDs being limited to 15 or fewer days per month.
- Tricyclic antidepressants are effective in preventing both tension-type headache and migraine headache and in the absence of contraindications should be considered first line. Start low and titrate slow realizing benefit can take up to 3 months.
- Behavioral strategies should be a part of any headache management plan.

DISCLOSURE

The authors have nothing to disclose.

REFERENCES

1. Finley CR, Chan DS, Garrison S, et al. What re the most common conditions in primary care? Can Fam Physician 2018;64:832–40.
2. GBD 2016 Headache Collaborators. Global, regional and national burden of migraine and tension-type headache, 1990-2016: a systematic analysis for the Global Burden of Disease Study 016. Lancet Neurol 2017;17(11):954–76.
3. Do TP, Remmers A, Schytz HW, et al. Red and orange flags for secondary headaches in clinical practice: SNNOOP10 list. Neurology 2019;92:134.
4. Martelli P, Birbeck GL, Katsarava Z, et al. The Global Burden of Disease survey 2010: lifting the burden and thinking outside-the-box on headache disorders. J Headache Pain 2013;14:13.
5. Schartz BS, Stewart WF, Simon D, et al. Epidemiology of tension-type headache. JAMA 1998;279:381.
6. Jensen R. Peripheral and central mechanism in tension-type headache: an update. Cephalalgia 2003;23(Supple 1):49.
7. Rasmussen BK. Epidemiology of headache. Cephalalgia 1995;15:45.
8. Moore Ra, Derry S, Wiffen PJ, et al. Evidence for the efficacy of acute treatment of episodic tension-type headache: methodological critique of randomized trials for oral treatments. Pain 2014;155:2220.
9. Verhagen AP, Damen L, Berger MY, et al. Lack of benefit for prophylactic drugs of tension-type headache in adults: a systematic review. Fam Pract 2010;27:151.
10. Jacson JL, Mancuso JM, Nickoloff S, et al. Tricyclic and tetracyclic antidepressants for the prevention of frequent episodic or chronic tension-type headaches

in adults: a systematic review and meta-analysis. J Gen Intern Med 2017;32: 1351.

11. Lenaerts ME. Pharmacoprophylaxis of tension-type headache. Curr Pain Headache Rep 2005;9:442.

12. Lampl C, Marecek S, May A, et al. A prospective, open-label, long-term study of the efficacy and tolerability of topiramate in the prophylaxis of chronic tension-type headache. Cephalalgia 2006;26:1203.

13. Gobel H, Hamouz V, Hansen C, et al. Chronic tension type headaches: amitriptyline reduces clinical headache-duration and experimental pain sensitivity but does not alter pericranial muscle activity readings. Pain 1994;59:241.

14. Karadas O, Gul HL, Inan LE. Lidocaine injection of pericranial myofascial trigger points in the treatment of frequent episodic tension-type headache. J Headache Pain 2013;14:44.

15. Jackson JL, Kuriyama A, Hayashino Y. Botulinum toxin A for prophylactic treatment of migraine and tension headaches in adults: a meta-analysis. JAMA 2012;307:1736.

16. Penzien DB, Rains JC, Lipchik GL, et al. Behavioral interventions for tension-type headache: overview of current therapies and recommendations for a self-management model for chronic headache. Curr Pain Headache Rep 2004;8:489.

17. Nestoriuc Y, Rief W, Martin A. Meta-analysis of biofeedback for tension-type headache: efficacy, specificity, and treatment moderators. J Consult Clin Psychol 2008;76:379.

18. Holrod KA, O'Donnell FJ, Stensland M, et al. Management of chronic tension type headache with tricyclic antidepressant medication, stress management therapy, and their combination: a randomized controlled trial. JAMA 2001;285:2208.

19. Abbott RB, Hui K, Hayes R, et al. A randomized trial of Tai Chi for tension headaches. Evid Based Complement Alternat Med 2007;4(1):107.

20. Kim S. Effects of yoga exercises for headaches: a systematic review of randomized controlled trials. J Phys Ther Sci 2015;27:2377.

21. Chaibi A, Russell MB. Manual therapies for primary chronic headaches: a systematic review of randomized controlled trials. J Headache Pain 2014;15:67.

22. Charles A. Vasodilation out of the picture as a cause of migraine headache. Lancet Neurol 2013;12:419.

23. Cutrer FM. Pathophysiology of migraine. Semin Neurol 2006;26:171.

24. Hamel E. Serotonin and migraine: biology and clinical implications. Cephalalgia 2007;27:1293.

25. Panconesi A. Serotonin and migraine: a reconsideration of the central theory. J Headache Pain 2008;9:267.

26. Lance JVV, Anthony M. Some clinical aspects of migraine. A prospective survey of 500 patients. Arch Neurol 1966;15:356.

27. Charles A. The evolution of a migraine attack—a review of recent evidence. Headache 2013;53:413.

28. Barbanti P, Fabgrini G, Pesare M, et al. Unilateral cranial autonomic symptoms in migraine. Cephalalgia 2002;22:256.

29. Rapoport AM, Bigal ME. ID-migraine. Neurol Sci 2004;25 Supple 3:S258.

30. Cousins G, Hijazze S, Van de Laar FA, et al. Diagnostic accuracy of the ID Migraine: a systematic review and meta-analysis. Headache 2011;51.

31. Niere K. The presence of four simple history features can diagnosis migraine accurately. Australian J of Physiology 2006;52(4):304.

32. Maizels M, Burchette R. Rapid and sensitive paradigm for screening patients with headache in primary care settings. Headache 2003;43:441.

33. Derry S, Moore RA. Paracetamol (acetaminophen) with or without an antiemetic for acute migraine headaches in adults. Cochrane Database Syst Rev 2013;(4):CD008040.
34. Lipton RB, Steward WF, Ryan RE Jr, et al. Efficacy and safety of acetaminophen, aspirin, and caffeine in alleviating migraine headache pain; three double blind, randomized, placebo-controlled trials. Arch Neurol 1998;55:210.
35. Tfelt-Hansen P, Knight YE, Goadsby PJ. Triptans in migraine; a comparative review of pharmacology, pharmacokinetics and efficacy. Drugs 2000;60:1259.
36. Ferrari MD, Roon KL, Lipton RB, et al. Oral triptans (serotonin 5-HT (1B/1D) agonists) in acute migraine treatment: a meta-analysis of 53 trials. Lancet 2001; 358:1668.
37. Roberto G, Raschi E, Piccinni C, et al. Adverse cardiovascular events associated with triptans and ergotamines for treatment of migraine: systematic review of observational studies. Cephalalgia 2015;35:118.
38. Jamieson DG. The safety of triptans in the treatment of patients with migraine. Am J Med 2002;112:135.
39. Evans RW. Concomitant triptan and SSRI or SNRI use: what is the risk for serotonin syndrome? Headache 2008;42:1692.
40. Colman I, Friedman BW, Brown MD, et al. Parenteral dexamethasone for acute severe migraine headaches: meta-analysis of randomized controlled trials for preventing recurrence. BMJ 2008;336:1359.
41. MacGregor EA. In the clinic. Migraine. Ann Intern Med 2013;159:ITC5.
42. Kelman L. The triggers or precipitants of the acute migraine attack. Cephalalgia 2007;27:394.
43. Goadsby PJ, Lipton RB, Ferrari MD. Migraine—current understanding and treatment. N Engl J Med 2002;346:257.
44. Silberstein SD, Holland S, Freitag F, et al. Evidence-based guideline update: pharmacologic treatment for episodic migraine prevention in adults: report of the Quality Standards Subcommittee of the American Academy of Neurology and the American Headache Society. Neurology 2012;78:1337.
45. Reuter U, Goadsby PJ, Lanteri-Minet M, et al. Efficacy and tolerability of erenumab in patients with episodic migraine in whom two-to-four previous preventive treatments were unsuccessful: a randomized, double-blind, placebo-controlled phase 3b study. Lancet 2018;392:2280.

A Case-Based Approach to Constipation in Primary Care

David B. Snell, MD[a],*, Saamia Faruqui, MD[a], Brian P. Bosworth, MD[b]

KEYWORDS

- Constipation • Defecatory disorder • Fiber • Laxatives • Anorectal manometry

KEY POINTS

- The rectal examination is the most important aspect of the physical examination in the evaluation of constipation.
- Colonoscopy should be considered in patients with warning symptoms, with iron deficiency anemia, and meeting criteria for age-appropriate colorectal cancer screening.
- Fiber and laxatives are the backbone of initial treatment.
- If fiber and laxatives fail, there are multiple effective and safe second-line therapies.
- Patients with refractory symptoms or high suspicion of a defecatory disorder should be referred to a gastroenterologist for anorectal manometry and balloon expulsion testing.

Constipation is a commonly encountered problem in primary care. Although the initial evaluation and treatment have common threads, certain points of emphasis in the history and physical examination can help formulate a targeted diagnostic and treatment plan. This approach is explored using a series of patient cases to illustrate particular points in the evaluation of a patient with chronic constipation.

INTRODUCTORY CASE: NORMAL/SLOW-TRANSIT CONSTIPATION, PART 1

A 62-year-old woman with hypothyroidism and hypertension presents with several months of constipation. She passes 1 hard, lumpy bowel movement every other day, occasionally with straining. She denies changes in her weight, nausea, vomiting, abdominal pain, melena, or hematochezia. She has not yet tried any medications. Her hypertension is well controlled on amlodipine. She denies any prior abdominal surgeries or family history of colorectal cancer. Her diet consists of 1 to 2 servings of fruits and vegetables daily.

[a] Division of Gastroenterology & Hepatology, Department of Medicine, New York University, 550 First Avenue, New York, NY 10016, USA; [b] Department of Medicine, New York University, 550 First Avenue, HCC 3-15, New York, NY 10016, USA
* Corresponding author. 550 First Avenue, New York, NY 10016.
E-mail address: David.Snell2@nyulangone.org

Med Clin N Am 105 (2021) 55–73
https://doi.org/10.1016/j.mcna.2020.08.015
0025-7125/21/© 2020 Elsevier Inc. All rights reserved.

Definition

Constipation encompasses a wide variety of patient-reported symptoms. Most patients commonly use terms, such as straining, hard stools, or inability to have a bowel movement.[1] The Rome IV criteria (**Box 1**) provide a consensus definition for functional chronic constipation.[2]

Although the irritable bowel syndrome constipation subtype may have similar symptoms, functional constipation is not characterized by abdominal pain. The diagnosis and management of the irritable bowel syndrome constipation subtype are not a focus of this article.

Normal Colonic Function

Understanding constipation requires knowledge of normal colonic physiology, including absorption, motor function, innervation, and defecatory function (**Box 2**).

Epidemiology

The overall prevalence of constipation is estimated at 14% but varies widely.[3] The cumulative incidence over a 12-year period was 17% in 1 large population study.[4]

Risk Factors

Risk factors for chronic constipation are listed in **Box 3**, with medications associated with constipation listed in **Box 4**.

Secondary Causes of Constipation

There also are several secondary causes of constipation (**Box 5**) that can be broken down broadly into mechanical obstruction, metabolic, neurologic, and myopathic disorders.

Effect on Quality of Life

Constipated patients, in particular the elderly, have greater psychological distress, depression, and anxiety and a lower sense of well-being.[5] They also experience lower levels of physical functioning and higher perception of bodily pain.[6]

Box 1
Rome IV diagnostic criteria for functional chronic constipation

1. Must include 2 or more of the following:
   a. Straining during greater than 25% of defecations
   b. Lumpy or hard stools greater than 25% of defecations
   c. Sensation of incomplete evacuation greater than 25% of defecations
   d. Sensation of anorectal blockage greater than 25% of defecations
   e. Manual maneuvers to facilitate greater than 25% of defecations (ie, inserting a finger into the rectum to remove stool or inserting a finger into the vagina to support the pelvic floor and ease defecation)
   f. Less than 3 defecations a week

2. Loose stools rarely are present without the use of laxatives

3. Insufficient criteria for irritable bowel syndrome

Criteria fulfilled for the last 3 months with symptom onset at least 6 months prior.

Adapted from Lacy B, Mearin F, Chang L, et al. Bowel Disorders. Gastroenterology 2016;150(6):1393-1407.

Box 2
Normal colonic function

Absorption

- Sodium and water are absorbed along an osmotic gradient, extracting greater than 90% of fluid coming from the small intestine

Motor function

- Purpose
  a. Delays passage of luminal contents to allow for absorption
  b. Allows for propulsion as well as storage of feces
- Consists of low-amplitude and high-amplitude propagated contractions

Innervation

- Under control of the enteric nervous system, regulated by the interstitial cells of Cajal, which act as pacemakers

Defecatory function

- Urge to defecate occurs when mechanoreceptors in the upper anal canal sense distention.
- Contraction of abdominal muscles raises intrapelvic pressure.
- Simultaneously, the puborectalis muscle relaxes, causing descent of the pelvic floor and straightening of the anorectal angle.
- Internal anal sphincter also relaxes under parasympathetic control from S2.
- Relaxation of the external anal sphincter allows for stool expulsion.

Data from Lembo AJ. Constipation. In: Lembo M, Friedman LS, Sleisenger MH. Sleisenger & Fordtran's gastrointestinal and liver disease: pathophysiology, diagnosis, management. Philadelphia: Saunders; 2002. p. 270-96.

Younger patients are affected predominantly by decreased social and mental well-being, especially women.[7] The magnitude of the impact on health-related quality of life is comparable to other common, chronic conditions, such as allergies, diabetes, and stable inflammatory bowel disease.[8]

Health Care Burden

The physical and mental impairments resulting from chronic constipation can lead to work absenteeism and impairment as well as increased resource utilization and costs.[9]

Box 3
Constipation risk factors

- Older age
- Female gender
- Nonwhite ethnicity
- Low socioeconomic status
- Low level of education
- Low level of physical activity

Adapted from Lembo AJ. Constipation. In: Lembo M, Friedman LS, Sleisenger MH. Sleisenger & Fordtran's gastrointestinal and liver disease: pathophysiology, diagnosis, management. Philadelphia: Saunders; 2002. p. 270-96.

> **Box 4**
> **Medications associated with constipation**
>
> - Acetaminophen
> - Aluminum-containing antacids
> - Anticholinergics
> - Anticonvulsants
> - Antiparkinsonian agents
> - Antipsychotics
> - Antispasmodics
> - Calcium and iron supplements
> - Calcium channel blockers
> - Diuretics
> - Nonsteroidal anti-inflammatory drugs
> - Mu-opioid agonists
> - Tricyclic antidepressants
>
> *Adapted from* Lembo AJ. Constipation. In: Lembo M, Friedman LS, Sleisenger MH. Sleisenger & Fordtran's gastrointestinal and liver disease: pathophysiology, diagnosis, management. Philadelphia: Saunders; 2002. p. 270-96.

A third to half of outpatient visits for constipation are managed by a primary care provider, whereas only 14% are managed by a gastroenterologist.[10] Therefore, the diagnostic work-up and treatment plan fall largely on the primary care physician.

One study estimated the direct annual health care costs per patient at $7522, with individual out-of-pocket expenses of $390.[11] The annual direct costs to the health care system total $1.6 billion, with indirect costs of $140 million.[12]

Clinical questions for introductory case:

1. What are the key elements of the history and physical examination?
2. What laboratory tests should be considered?
3. What is the role of colonoscopy?
4. What first-line treatments should be recommended?

History

This case highlights key elements in the history. The first goal is to define clearly what the patient means by constipation. Symptoms of straining, lumpy or hard stools, sensation of incomplete evacuation or anorectal blockage, fewer than 3 bowel movements per week, and the use of manual maneuvers to facilitate defecation are key features to elicit. Symptoms of abdominal pain, bloating, or distention should prompt consideration of alternate etiologies, such as irritable bowel syndrome.[13] In all cases, the physician should inquire about alarm symptoms, including unintentional weight loss, severe abdominal pain, refractory nausea and vomiting, melena, and hematochezia. Rapid symptom onset is concerning.[1] If any of these features is present, further diagnostic work-up is needed.

Medical history should be queried for systemic disorders that could be secondary causes of constipation. A comprehensive review of prescribed and over-the-counter medications can identify medication-related causes. An early family history of

---

Box 5
Secondary causes of constipation

Mechanical obstruction

- Anal stenosis
- Colorectal cancer or stricture
- Extrinsic colonic compression
- Rectocele

Metabolic disorders

- Diabetes mellitus
- Hypercalcemia
- Hypokalemia
- Pregnancy
- Thyroid disease

Neurologic/myopathic disorders

- Amyloidosis
- Autonomic neuropathy
- Dermatomyositis
- Intestinal pseudo-obstruction
- Multiple sclerosis
- Parkinsonism
- Spinal cord injury
- Stroke
- Systemic sclerosis

Adapted from Lembo AJ. Constipation. In: Lembo M, Friedman LS, Sleisenger MH. Sleisenger & Fordtran's gastrointestinal and liver disease: pathophysiology, diagnosis, management. Philadelphia: Saunders; 2002. p. 270-96.

---

colorectal cancer may necessitate early colorectal cancer screening. Finally, a dietary and exercise history can assist in identifying lifestyle habits that can be altered to mitigate constipation.

Physical Examination

A general physical examination is unremarkable. Rectal examination is notable for no anal fissures or hemorrhoids, no stool in the rectal vault, no masses palpated, and normal resting anal sphincter tone and augmentation with simulated defecation.

The general physical examination may help uncover secondary causes of constipation. The rectal examination is the single most important aspect of the physical examination. Another case delves into the techniques and information gained from a thorough rectal examination.

Laboratory Work-up

The patient reports no recent laboratory testing, abdominopelvic imaging, or colonoscopy.

In the absence of other symptoms and signs, the only laboratory test necessary is a complete blood cell count to look for anemia.[13] If anemia is present, iron studies should be ordered, particularly if the anemia is microcytic. Iron deficiency anemia should prompt endoscopic evaluation in all men and postmenopausal women. If symptoms suggest a systemic disorder, it also is reasonable to check glucose, calcium, and thyroid function tests, but these are not recommended routinely.

A complete blood cell count, basic metabolic panel, and thyroid-stimulating hormone are normal.

When to Consult a Gastroenterologist: Colonoscopy

A gastroenterologist should be consulted for consideration of a colonoscopy if alarm symptoms or iron deficiency anemia are present.[14] Additionally, those who need age-appropriate colorectal cancer screening should undergo fecal immunochemical testing (FIT) or colonoscopy.[15] Colonoscopy should not be recommended routinely in patients without alarm features who have had age-appropriate colorectal cancer screening. A meta-analysis demonstrated no increase in colorectal cancer in patients with chronic constipation.[16] The diagnostic yield of colonoscopy in chronic constipation is low and comparable to the asymptomatic general population.[17]

Because she is at average risk, the patient is offered age-appropriate colorectal cancer screening with colonoscopy or FIT. The patient decides on annual FIT and subsequent testing is negative.

Treatment: Lifestyle and Risk Factor Modification

Constipation management starts with identification and modification of risk factors as well as nonpharmacologic measures. Patients should set aside unhurried, regular time for defecation, particularly after eating, in order to take advantage of physiologically increased colonic motility. Those who have difficulty expelling stool can try a support of at least 6 in under their feet so that their hips are flexed in a squatting position. Sedentary patients may benefit from increased physical activity.[18] Dehydration may worsen constipation, but there are no data showing that increased fluid intake improves constipation.[18] If feasible, medications with constipation as a side effect should be discontinued or switched.[13]

The patient is counseled on the lifestyle modifications, discussed previously, and her calcium channel blocker is switched to an alternative antihypertensive.

Treatment: Fiber

Increased fiber intake through diet and supplementation is the backbone of constipation treatment. Fiber bulks colonic residue, which improves colonic transit and stool consistency. Patients need a minimum of 20 g to 25 g of fiber daily, up to 38 g daily for men.[19] Whole-wheat starches, unrefined cereals, and fruits and vegetables contain the most dietary fiber. Dietary fiber alone can be effective in relieving mild constipation.[20]

If additional fiber is needed, there are several supplements commonly available (**Table 1**). These are made up primarily of soluble fiber, which has been shown to improve constipation.[21] Most are available as a powder or pill, with an onset of action of 1 day to 3 days. A starting dose of 4 g to 6 g daily is appropriate for most formulations. Fiber should be taken with adequate liquid and at least an hour apart from other medications. Physicians should advise patients to increase fiber gradually over several weeks because fiber can cause bloating and flatulence, which can lead to poor adherence.[19] Fiber should be avoided in those with gastrointestinal strictures or obstruction.

Table 1
Common fiber supplements

Fiber	Efficacy/Side Effects
Psyllium	• Improves stool frequency,[22] straining, pain on defecation, and stool consistency[21] • Effective in 85% of those without a defecatory disorder or slow-transit constipation[20] • May increase bloating
Methylcellulose	• Improves stool frequency but not consistency or ease of passage[23] • Less likely to cause bloating[23]
Polycarbophil	• Improves ease of stool passage[24] • Less likely to cause bloating[23]
Wheat dextrin	• May increase bloating

Data from Refs.[20-24]

The patient is counseled to increase her intake of whole grains and vegetables and also to add psyllium, 4 g to 6 g daily, with slow up-titration over a 2-week period.

These measures result in 50% improvement in her symptoms. She asks what else can be done to further alleviate her constipation.

Treatment: Laxatives

If fiber supplementation is not tolerated or does not adequately relieve constipation, then laxatives should be added. Osmotic laxatives work by drawing fluid into the lumen of the colon. Stimulant laxatives alter electrolyte transport and increase motor activity. Osmotic and stimulant laxatives are both effective, with a number needed to treat (NNT) of 3, although there are no direct comparisons.[25] Generally, osmotic laxatives are more well tolerated, and stimulant laxatives work more quickly. Therefore, osmotic laxatives should be used primarily for maintenance therapy, and stimulant laxatives work well as rescue therapy. Stool softeners and emollients can help lubricate hard stools by acting as surfactants and emulsifiers, respectively. They should be used sparingly, however, due to a lack of established efficacy. Based on ease of administration, oral laxatives are preferable to suppositories or enemas for mild to moderate constipation. Common oral laxatives are described in **Table 2**.

Those patients with severe constipation or a defecatory disorder may benefit from the addition of rectally administered laxatives. Suppositories are best administered 30 minutes after breakfast to take advantage of physiologic increases in colonic motility. In cases of fecal impaction, mineral oil enemas are particularly helpful after manual disimpaction. Long-term use of suppositories and enemas may lead to rectal mucosal irritation. Common rectal laxatives are described in **Table 3**.

The patient is prescribed once-daily polyethylene glycol. She is advised to add oral bisacodyl as needed. With these interventions, she reports complete relief of her symptoms within 1 week.

CLINICS CARE POINTS

- Clearly define what the patient means by constipation
- In all patients, elicit warning symptoms that should prompt additional evaluation
- The rectal examination is the single most important aspect of the physical examination

Table 2
Common oral laxatives

Oral Laxative	Typical Dosage	Onset of Action	Efficacy	Side Effects
Osmotic				
Polyethylene glycol	17–34 g, once or twice daily	1–4 d	Improves stool frequency and consistency with complete, long-term remission in most[22,26] More effective than lactulose for improving stool frequency and consistency, abdominal pain, and decreasing need for other agents[27]	Mild abdominal bloating and cramps[26]
Lactulose	15–30 mL, once or twice daily	1–2 d	Improves stool frequency[22]	Abdominal distention, discomfort, and flatulence
Magnesium hydroxide	15–30 mL, once or twice daily	1–6 h	May improve stool frequency and consistency[28]	Fluid shifts in advanced renal and cardiac disease[28]
Stimulant				
Bisacodyl	5–10 mg, daily	6–24 h	Improves stool frequency, consistency, straining, and sensation of obstruction[29] Improves constipation related quality-of-life metrics[29]	Abdominal cramping and pain, 20% discontinue[29] No evidence chronic use leads to structural or functional colonic impairment[30]
Senna	7.5–15 mg, daily	6–12 h	Few data to support	Abdominal cramps No evidence chronic use leads to structural or functional colonic impairment[30]
Stool softener				
Docusate	100 mg, twice daily	1–3 d	Less effective than psyllium[31] Minimal, if any, benefit[28]	Well tolerated
Emollient				
Mineral oil	5–15 mL, daily	6–8 h	No data in adults	Lipoid pneumonia, fat-soluble vitamin malabsorption, anal seepage[19]

Data from Refs.[19,22,26–31]

Table 3 Common rectal laxatives		
Rectal Laxative	**Onset of Action**	**Side Effects[a]**
Suppositories		
Glycerin Bisacodyl	15–60 min	• Bisacodyl may be more effective
Enemas		
Phosphate	2–15 min	• Hyperphosphatemia/hypocalcemia (avoid in advanced renal disease)
Saline		• Lowest chance of electrolyte abnormalities or mucosal irritation
Tap water Soapsuds		• In large volume, causes electrolyte abnormalities (avoid in advanced renal or cardiac disease) • Tap water less likely to cause mucosal irritation
Mineral oil	6–8 h	• May cause anal seepage

[a] *Data from* Lembo AJ. Constipation. In: Lembo M, Friedman LS, Sleisenger MH. Sleisenger & Fordtran's gastrointestinal and liver disease: pathophysiology, diagnosis, management. Philadelphia: Saunders; 2002. p. 270-96.

- A complete blood cell count is the only universally indicated laboratory test. Other testing should be guided by the history and physical examination.
- Colonoscopy should be considered in patients with warning symptoms, with iron deficiency anemia, and meeting criteria for age-appropriate colorectal cancer screening.
- Fiber is the backbone of initial treatment.
- If fiber is not tolerated or inadequate, then maintenance therapy with osmotic laxatives and rescue therapy with stimulant laxatives should be used.

CASE: NORMAL/SLOW-TRANSIT CONSTIPATION, PART 2

The patient returns in 6 months with worsening constipation. She has been compliant with the treatments previously discussed. Now, however, she is not experiencing complete relief of her symptoms. Aside from worsening stool frequency and straining, there are no new symptoms, including no new alarm symptoms. There are no changes in her physical examination. She asks what other treatment options are available.

Clinical question:

1. What second-line treatments are available if fiber and laxatives are inadequate?

In those with constipation refractory to fiber as well as osmotic and stimulant laxatives, pharmacologic therapy with an oral secretagogue or prokinetic is the next step. Secretagogues, such as a chloride channel activator and guanylate cyclase agonists, increase intestinal fluid secretion, which improves constipation. A serotonin–5-hydroxytryptamine$_4$ agonist works as a prokinetic by increasing colonic motility. Second-line therapies are described in **Table 4**.

The patient is started on lubiprostone with complete resolution of symptoms.

CLINICS CARE POINT

- If fiber and laxatives are inadequate, there are multiple secretagogues and a prokinetic that can be used as second-line therapy

Table 4
Second-line medications

Medication	Typical Administration	Onset of Action	Efficacy	Side Effects
Chloride channel activator				
Lubiprostone	24 µg, twice daily (with food)	1–2 d	Improves stool frequency, consistency, and straining[32]; NNT 4[25]	Dose adjust in advanced cirrhosis Nausea, headache, diarrhea[32]
Guanylate cyclase C agonists				
Linaclotide	145 µg, once daily (before breakfast)	12–24 h	Improves stool frequency, consistency, straining, bloating and abdominal discomfort; NNT 6[33]	Diarrhea, 4% discontinue[33]
Plecanatide	3 mg, once daily	12–24 h	Improves stool frequency, consistency, straining, and abdominal discomfort[34]	Well tolerated
Serotonin–5-hydroxytryptamine$_4$ agonist				
Prucalopride	2 mg, once daily		Improves stool frequency, satisfaction with bowel movements[35]; NNT 6[25]	Dose adjust for renal impairment Headache, abdominal pain, nausea, diarrhea[35]

Data from Refs.[25,32–35]

CASE: DEFECATORY DISORDER, PART 1

A 31-year-old woman with depression and anxiety presents with several months of constipation. She describes prolonged straining and a sensation of incomplete evacuation, sometimes requiring manual removal of stool from her rectum. She reports no alarm symptoms. She has had 3 vaginal deliveries and a history of physical abuse. There is no family history of colorectal cancer. She has not yet tried any medications.

On inspection, the rectal examination is notable for external hemorrhoids and no anal fissures or rectal prolapse. The anocutaneous reflex is intact. On digital rectal examination, there is soft brown stool in the rectal vault, no masses or stricture, and high resting anal sphincter tone with inappropriate descent of the perineum and examiner's finger during simulated defecation. The rest of the general physical examination is unremarkable.

A complete blood cell count is normal.

Clinical questions:

1. What elements in the history and physical examination suggest a defecatory disorder?
2. What are the important aspects of a thorough rectal examination?
3. What is the initial treatment strategy in defecatory disorders?

History

There are several clues that suggest a defecatory disorder. Common symptoms include excessive straining, incomplete evacuation, fewer than 3 bowel movements weekly, and use of manual maneuvers.[36] A quarter of patients report a history of sexual or physical abuse.[36] Depression and anxiety are frequent comorbidities. Obstetric and surgical histories can provide insight into possible anatomic reasons for a defecatory disorder.

The Rectal Examination

A thorough visual and digital rectal examination (described in **Box 6**) is able to identify a defecatory disorder, with 75% sensitivity and 85% specificity.[37] A normal rectal examination does not exclude a defecatory disorder.

Pathophysiology of Defecatory Disorders

Defecatory disorders arise from a failure to coordinate the abdominal, anorectal, and pelvic floor muscles. Usually this is due to inappropriate contraction of the anal sphincter and/or an inability to adequately raise intrarectal pressure.[1] Rarely, there is a structural abnormality, such as a rectocele or rectal prolapse. At least 25% of patients with functional constipation have a defecatory disorder.[38]

Treatment

The initial treatment strategy is similar to the introductory case. The patient first should be counseled on lifestyle and risk factor modification. Pharmacotherapy involves fiber and laxatives as first-line treatment.

The patient is advised to get a footstool to use while sitting on the toilet and is started on fiber and oral laxatives with improvement in her symptoms.

Box 6
Steps of a rectal examination

1. Place the patient in the left lateral position with the hips flexed.

2. Visualize the anus and surrounding area: look for rectal prolapse, anal fissures, and external hemorrhoids.

3. Test perianal sensation and the anocutaneous reflex (contraction of the perianal skin with light pinprick or scratch) in order to screen for neuromuscular disorders.

4. Perform digital palpation and maneuvers to assess anorectal function
   a. Gently place a lubricated and gloved finger into the rectum to assess for fecal impaction, rectal stricture, rectal prolapse, rectal mass, internal hemorrhoids, and resting anal sphincter tone.
   b. Ask the patient to squeeze the examiner's inserted finger to assess anal sphincter tone.
   c. Place left hand over the patient's abdomen while asking the patient to bear down as if having a bowel movement. This allows for assessment of push effort, ability to relax the anal sphincter, and degree of perineal descent.
   d. If the patient is unable to contract the abdominal muscles sufficiently, unable to relax the anal sphincter, exhibits a paradoxic contraction of the anal sphincter, or has inappropriate perineal descent (<1 cm or >4 cm), then these are suggestive of a defecatory disorder.

Data from Tantiphlachiva K, Rao P, Attaluri A, Rao SS. Digital rectal examination is a useful tool for identifying patients with dyssynergia. Clin Gastroenterol Hepatol 2010;8(11):955-60.

CLINICS CARE POINTS

- Excessive straining, incomplete evacuation, few spontaneous bowel movements, and use of manual maneuvers to expel stool are typical features of a defecatory disorder.
- The rectal examination can be highly useful in determining suspicion for a defecatory disorder.
- Even in those with high suspicion for a defecatory disorder, the initial treatment should consist of lifestyle modifications, fiber, and laxatives.

CASE: DEFECATORY DISORDER, PART 2

The patient returns 3 months later reporting that she still is straining with a sense of incomplete evacuation. She has required bisacodyl suppositories in addition to oral laxatives to try to stimulate bowel movements. She asks if there is anything further that can be done.

Clinical questions:

1. What is the role of anorectal manometry, balloon expulsion testing, and defecography?
2. What treatment is most effective in defecatory disorders?

When to Consult a Gastroenterologist: Ancillary Testing

Because the history and rectal examination findings are typical of a defecatory disorder and fiber and laxatives have been ineffective, referral to a gastroenterologist for ancillary testing is indicated. Anorectal manometry and the balloon expulsion test can confirm the presence of a defecatory disorder that may be amenable to biofeedback therapy. The challenge resides in access to subspecialists who perform these tests and physical therapists who are trained in biofeedback. If these resources are not readily available, then it is reasonable to initially pursue treatment with first-line and second-line therapies even if a defecatory disorder is strongly suspected.

Anorectal manometry assesses the resting and squeeze pressure of the anal sphincter as well as the relaxation of the anal sphincter during straining.[39] Normally, there should be an increase in intrarectal pressure and decrease in anal sphincter pressure. Inappropriate contraction of the anal sphincter while bearing down is the hallmark of a defecatory disorder.

The balloon expulsion test involves rectal insertion of a balloon, which then is inflated with saline. Inability to expel the balloon within 1 minute is 88% to 89% sensitive and specific for a defecatory disorder, with a negative predictive value of 97%.[40] Imaging with defecography plays an adjunctive role by evaluating for anatomic abnormalities and providing additional information when anorectal testing results are inconclusive or inconsistent.[13]

The patient is referred for anorectal manometry and balloon expulsion testing. Anorectal manometry is notable for inadequate relaxation of resting anal sphincter pressure and a paradoxic increase in pressure on simulated defecation. Balloon expulsion time is greater than 1 minute. She is diagnosed with a defecatory disorder and asks how this will alter treatment.

Treatment: biofeedback

Once a defecatory disorder has been confirmed, treatment with biofeedback should be implemented. Biofeedback utilizes a rectal catheter or electromyography in conjunction with a trained physical therapist to provide visual or auditory feedback regarding functioning of the anal sphincter and pelvic floor muscles. This improves pelvic floor muscle relaxation and coordination. The success rate of biofeedback is up to 70%.[41] Biofeedback increases stool frequency, decreases digital maneuvers, and improves satisfaction with bowel movements.[42]

The patient is referred to a physical therapist trained in biofeedback. After several weeks, she notes significant improvement in straining and sense of complete evacuation.

CLINICS CARE POINTS

- Patients with symptoms refractory to first-line and second-line therapies or with high suspicion of a defecatory disorder should be referred for anorectal manometry and balloon expulsion testing.
- If a defecatory disorder is confirmed, biofeedback is highly effective.

CASE: OPIOID-INDUCED CONSTIPATION

A 55-year-old man with chronic back pain and depression presents with constipation for the past few weeks. He describes small, hard, infrequent bowel movements. He reports no alarm symptoms. He follows with a pain management specialist and is on long-acting opioids. Recently, his dose of short-acting opioids was increased for breakthrough pain. He already is on polyethylene glycol daily.

Rectal examination is normal on visualization and notable for hard stool in the rectal vault on digital examination. General physical examination is unremarkable. His hemoglobin is normal, and he had a normal screening colonoscopy at age 50 years old.

Clinical question:

1. What is the treatment approach in opioid-induced constipation?

Opioid-Induced Constipation

Opioid-induced constipation is an increasingly common secondary cause of chronic constipation. Opioids cause constipation by slowing gut motility. Among patients using opioids, 40% have fewer than 3 bowel movements weekly despite 80% taking laxatives to prevent constipation.[43]

The patient is advised to increase fiber and add a stimulant laxative, but, despite these measures, he continues to have infrequent bowel movements. He then is started on lubiprostone, with 50% improvement. He wants to know what other therapies can be offered.

Treatment: Mu-opioid Antagonists

For many patients on opioids, increased fiber and laxatives can improve constipation. Lubiprostone also is effective.[44] In those with refractory symptoms, peripheral mu-opioid antagonists (**Table 5**) can be useful. These act selectively in the gut to reverse opioid-mediated dysmotility. All maintenance laxatives should be discontinued prior to initiation of these medications. If symptom response is not optimal after 3 days, then laxatives may be reintroduced. All mu-opioid antagonists are contraindicated in the setting of gastrointestinal obstruction.

The patient's laxative regimen is discontinued, and he is started on oral methylnaltrexone. He notes improved bowel movement frequency within 3 days.

CLINICS CARE POINT

- The initial treatments of opioid-induced constipation include fiber, laxatives, and lubiprostone. If refractory, peripherally acting mu-opioid antagonists should be used

CASE: SEVERELY REFRACTORY CONSTIPATION

A 60-year-old woman with diabetes and depression presents with several years of constipation. She describes 1 to 2 hard stools weekly with straining and a sense of incomplete evacuation. She denies alarm symptoms. She has seen several physicians for these symptoms and has tried fiber, laxatives, and multiple second-line therapies. Additionally, she once was referred to a gastroenterologist for anorectal manometry and balloon expulsion testing, with inconsistent results. Then she underwent magnetic resonance defecography, which did not show any anatomic abnormalities or findings consistent with a defecatory disorder. She requested a trial of biofeedback therapy but did not have significant improvement after several weeks. She wants to know which specialists she should see regarding next steps.

Rectal examination and general physical examination are unremarkable. Her laboratory test results are normal. She had a normal colonoscopy 1 year ago for screening.

Clinical questions:

1. What is the role of colonic transit studies?
2. When should a surgeon be consulted for refractory constipation?

When to Consult a Gastroenterologist: Role of Colonic Transit Studies

Patients who have failed first-line and second-line treatments and do not have a defecatory disorder should have a colonic transit study to determine whether slow or normal-transit constipation is present. Colonic transit studies also be should considered in patients who do not respond to biofeedback.

Table 5
Peripherally acting mu-opioid antagonists

Medication	Typical Dosage	Efficacy	Side Effects
Methylnaltrexone	450 mg, once daily by mouth Or 12 mg, once daily subcutaneously	Oral form improves spontaneous bowel movement frequency[45] Subcutaneous form more efficacious than lubiprostone, prucalopride, naloxegol, oral methylnaltrexone[46]	Dose adjust with severe hepatic or renal impairment Highest frequency of side effects, such as abdominal pain, flatulence, and nausea
Naloxegol	25 mg, once daily	Improves spontaneous bowel movement frequency[47]	Avoid use with CYP3A4 inhibitors and in severe hepatic impairment Dose adjust with renal impairment
Naldemedine	0.2 mg, once daily	Improves spontaneous bowel movement frequency[48]	Avoid in severe hepatic impairment

Data from Refs.[45–48]

The 2 most common colonic transit studies are radiopaque markers and a wireless motility capsule. Radiopaque markers are ingested by the patient and abdominal radiography is completed after 5 days to assess the number of retained markers. Patients should maintain a high-fiber diet and avoid any laxatives prior. If more than 20% of the markers are retained throughout the colon, this can be consistent with slow-transit constipation.

Wireless motility capsules can assess motility disorders throughout the entire gastrointestinal tract. The capsule is swallowed and sends continuous temperature, pH, and pressure measurements. Normal colonic transit time using this capsule is less than 44 hours in men or 59 hours in women.[49] The wireless capsule is useful when patients are considered for colectomy because it also assesses upper gastrointestinal transit.[50] The capsule should not be used in patients with pacemakers or defibrillators, swallowing disorders, or suspected strictures or obstruction.

Pathophysiology of Slow-Transit and Normal-Transit Constipation

Slow-transit constipation is a result of disordered colonic motor function. Patients with more severe slow-transit constipation have fewer high-amplitude propagated contractions.[1] Patients with normal-transit constipation have physiologically normal colonic motor function. Among those with functional constipation, 13% have slow-transit constipation, 59% have normal-transit constipation, and 3% have a combination of slow-transit constipation and a defecatory disorder.[38]

The patient is referred to a gastroenterologist for a colonic transit study. She has a wireless motility capsule that shows a colonic transit time of 70 hours with normal upper gastrointestinal transit times and is diagnosed with slow-transit constipation. She asks about the next steps in treatment.

When to Consult a Surgeon

A surgeon should be consulted

1. If imaging demonstrates an anatomic etiology for a defecatory disorder
2. In severe refractory cases of slow-transit constipation and/or defecatory disorders

For example, if magnetic resonance defecography is compatible with a large rectocele, surgical repair should be considered. In those with a refractory defecatory disorder and/or slow-transit constipation, sacral nerve stimulation can be considered. This involves surgical implantation of a neuromodulator device in those who have failed laxatives and biofeedback. Sacral nerve stimulation can increase bowel movements and decrease straining and incomplete evacuation.[51]

Total colectomy with ileorectal anastomosis can improve severe refractory slow-transit constipation. Only patients who demonstrate objective evidence of slow-transit constipation without upper gastrointestinal dysmotility should be considered. Additionally, a defecatory disorder must be ruled out, and patients must undergo psychiatric evaluation. In the appropriate patient, surgery can improve quality of life.[38]

The patient is referred to a colorectal surgeon and a psychiatrist for evaluation. She is deemed a good candidate for total colectomy with ileorectal anastomosis, and after surgery, her symptoms are improved immensely.

CLINICS CARE POINTS

- Patients with medically refractory constipation who do not have a defecatory disorder or have a defecatory disorder that is nonresponsive to biofeedback should

be referred to a gastroenterologist for a colonic transit study to guide further management
- Patients with anatomic reasons for outlet obstruction or severe refractory cases of slow-transit constipation and/or defecatory disorders should be referred to a surgeon

SUMMARY

The case-based approach outlined in this article highlights commonly encountered scenarios and provides a road map for management. Fiber and laxatives are the backbone of initial therapy. Key elements in the history and physical examination can guide next steps in those with refractory symptoms and allow primary care physicians to make the proper referrals to specialists.

DISCLOSURE

The authors have nothing to disclose.

REFERENCES

1. Lembo AJ. Constipation. In: Lembo M, Friedman LS, Sleisenger MH, editors. Sleisenger & Fordtran's gastrointestinal and liver disease: pathophysiology, diagnosis, management. Philadelphia: Saunders; 2002. p. 270–96.
2. Lacy B, Mearin F, Chang L, et al. Bowel disorders. Gastroenterology 2016;150(6): 1393–407.
3. Suares NC, Ford AC. Prevalence of, and risk factors for, chronic idiopathic constipation in the community: Systematic review and meta-analysis. Am J Gastroenterol 2011;106:1582–91.
4. Choung RS, Locke GR 3rd, Schleck CD, et al. Cumulative incidence of chronic constipation: a population-based study 1988-2003. Aliment Pharmacol Ther 2007;26:1521–8.
5. Glia A, Lindberg G. Quality of life in patients with different types of functional constipation. Scand J Gastroenterol 1997;32(11):1083–9.
6. O'Keefe EA, Talley NJ, Tangalos EG, et al. A bowel symptom questionnaire for the elderly. J Gerontol 1992;47:M116–21.
7. Wald A, Scarpignato C, Kamm MA, et al. The burden of constipation on quality of life: results of a multinational survey. Aliment Pharmacol Ther 2007;26:227–36.
8. Belsey J, Greenfield S, Candy D, et al. Systematic review: impact of constipation on quality of life in adults and children. Aliment Pharmacol Ther 2010;31:938–49.
9. Sun SX, DiBonaventura M, Purayidathil FW, et al. Impact of chronic constipation on health-related quality of life, work productivity, and healthcare resource use: an analysis of the National Health and Wellness Survey. Dig Dis Sci 2011;56: 2688–95.
10. Shah ND, Chitkara DK, Locke GR, et al. Ambulatory care for constipation in the United States, 1993-2004. Am J Gastroenterol 2008;103:1746–53.
11. Nyrop KA, Palsson OS, Levy RL, et al. Costs of health care for irritable bowel syndrome, chronic constipation, functional diarrhoea and functional abdominal pain. Aliment Pharmacol Ther 2007;26:237–48.
12. Everhart JE, Ruhl CE. Burden of digestive diseases in the United States part I: Overall and upper gastrointestinal diseases. Gastroenterology 2009;136:376–86.

13. Bharucha AE, Dorn SD, Lembo A, et al. American Gastroenterological Association medical position statement on constipation. Gastroenterology 2013;144: 211–7.

14. Qureshi W, Adler DG, Davila RE, et al. ASGE guideline: guideline on the use of endoscopy in the management of constipation. Gastrointest Endosc 2005;62: 199–201.

15. Levin B, Lieberman DA, McFarland B, et al. Screening and surveillance for the early detection of colorectal cancer and adenomatous polyps, 2008: A joint guideline from the American Cancer Society, the US Multi-Society Task Force on Colorectal Cancer, and the American College of Radiology. Gastroenterology 2008;134:1570–95.

16. Power AM, Talley NJ, Ford AC. Association between constipation and colorectal cancer: systematic review and meta-analysis. Am J Gastroenterol 2013;108: 894–903.

17. Pepin C, Ladabaum U. The yield of lower endoscopy in patients with constipation: Survey of a university hospital, a public county hospital, and a Veterans Administration medical center. Gastrointest Endosc 2002;56:325–32.

18. Muller-Lissner SA, Kamm MA, Scarpignato C, et al. Myths and misconceptions about chronic constipation. Am J Gastroenterol 2005;100:232–42.

19. Lembo A, Camilleri M. Chronic constipation. N Engl J Med 2003;349:1360–8.

20. Voderholzer WA, Schatke W, Muhldorfer BE, et al. Clinical response to dietary fiber treatment of chronic constipation. Am J Gastroenterol 1997;92:95–8.

21. Suares NC, Ford AC. Systematic review: the effects of fibre in the management of chronic idiopathic constipation. Aliment Pharmacol Ther 2011;33:895–901.

22. Ramkumar D, Rao SS. Efficacy and safety of traditional medical therapies for chronic constipation: systematic review. Am J Gastroenterol 2005;100(4):936–71.

23. Hamilton J, Wagner J, Burdich B, et al. Clinical evaluation of methylcellulose as a bulk laxative. Dig Dis Sci 1988;33:993–8.

24. Toskes PP, Connery KL, Ritchey TW. Calcium polycarbophil compared with placebo in irritable bowel syndrome. Aliment Pharmacol Ther 1993;7:87–92.

25. Ford AD, Suarez ND. Effect of laxatives and pharmacological therapies in chronic idiopathic constipations: systematic review and meta-analysis. Gut 2011;60: 209–18.

26. Corazziari E, Badiali D, Bazzocchi G, et al. Long-term efficacy, safety, and tolerability of low daily doses of isosmotic polyethylene glycol electrolyte balanced solution (PMF-100) in the treatment of functional chronic constipation. Gut 2000;46: 522–6.

27. Lee-Robichaud H, Thomas K, Morgan J, et al. Lactulose vs polyethylene glycol for chronic constipation. Cochrane Database Syst Rev 2010;7:1–13.

28. American College of Gastroenterology Chronic Constipation Task Force. An evidence-based approach to the management of chronic constipation in North America. Am J Gastroenterol 2005;100:S1–4.

29. Kamm MA, Mueller-Lissner S, Wald A, et al. Oral bisacodyl is effective and well-tolerated in patients with chronic constipation. Clin Gastroenterol Hepatol 2011; 9(7):577–83.

30. Wald A. Is chronic use of stimulant laxatives harmful to the colon? J Clin Gastroenterol 2003;36(5):386–9.

31. McRorie JW, Daggy BP, Morel JG, et al. Psyllium is superior to docusate sodium for treatment of chronic constipation. Aliment Pharmacol Ther 1998;12:491–7.

32. Barish CF, Drossman D, Johanson JF, et al. Efficacy and safety of lubiprostone in patients with chronic constipation. Dig Dis Sci 2010;55:1090–7.

33. Lembo AJ, Schneier HA, Shiff SJ, et al. Two randomized trials of linaclotide for chronic constipation. N Engl J Med 2011;365:527–36.
34. Shailubhai K, Barrow L, Talluto C, et al. Plecanatide, a guanylate cyclase C agonist, improves bowel habits and symptoms associated with chronic constipation in a phase IIa clinical study. Am J Gastroenterol 2011;106:1316.
35. Camilleri M, Kerstens R, Rykx A, et al. A placebo-controlled trial of prucalopride for severe chronic constipation. N Engl J Med 2008;358:2344–54.
36. Rao SS, Tuteja AK, Vellema T, et al. Dyssynergic defecation: Demographics, symptoms, stool patterns, and quality of life. J Clin Gastroenterol 2004;38:680–5.
37. Tantiphlachiva K, Rao P, Attaluri A, et al. Digital rectal examination is a useful tool for identifying patients with dyssynergia. Clin Gastroenterol Hepatol 2010;8(11):955–60.
38. Nyam DC, Pemberton JH, Ilstrup DM, et al. Long-term results of surgery for chronic constipation. Dis Colon Rectum 1997;40(3):273–9.
39. Rao S, Patel R. How useful are manometric tests of anorectal function in the management of defecation disorders? Am J Gastroenterol 1997;92:469–75.
40. Minguez M, Herreros B, Sanchiz V, et al. Predictive value of the balloon expulsion test for excluding the diagnosis of pelvic floor dyssynergia in constipation. Gastroenterology 2004;126:57–62.
41. Koh CE, Young CJ, Young JM, et al. Systematic review of randomized controlled trials of the effectiveness of biofeedback for pelvic floor dysfunction. Br J Surg 2008;95(9):1079–87.
42. Rao SS, Seaton K, Miller M, et al. Randomized controlled trial of biofeedback, sham feedback, and standard therapy for dyssynergic defecation. Clin Gastroenterol Hepatol 2007;5:331–8.
43. Pappagallo M. Incidence, prevalence, and management of opioid bowel dysfunction. Am J Surg 2001;182:11S–8S.
44. Jamal MM, Adams AB, Jansen JP, et al. A randomized, placebo-controlled trial of lubiprostone for opioid-induced constipation in chronic noncancer pain. Am J Gastroenterol 2015;110(5):725–32.
45. Rauck R, Slatkin NE, Stambler N, et al. Randomized, double-blind trial of oral methylnaltrexone for the treatment of opioid-induced constipation in patients with chronic noncancer pain. Pain Pract 2017;17(6):820–8.
46. Sridharan K, Sivaramakrishnan G. Drugs for treating opioid-induced constipation: A mixed treatment comparison network meta-analysis of randomized controlled clinical trials. J Pain Symptom Manage 2018;55:468–79.
47. Chey WD, Webster L, Sostek M, et al. Naloxegol for opioid-induced constipation in patients with noncancer pain. N Engl J Med 2014;370(25):2387–96.
48. Hale M, Wild J, Reddy J, et al. Naldemedine versus placebo for opioid-induced constipation (COMPOSE-1 and COMPOSE-2): two multicentre, phase 3, double-blind, randomised, parallel-group trials. Lancet Gastroenterol Hepatol 2017;2(8):555–64.
49. Rao SS, Kuo B, McCallum RW, et al. Investigation of colonic and whole-gut transit with wireless motility capsule and radiopaque markers in constipation. Clin Gastroenterol Hepatol 2009;7:537–44.
50. Glia A, Akerlund JE, Lindberg G. Outcome of colectomy for slow-transit constipation in relation to presence of small-bowel dysmotility. Dis Colon Rectum 2004;47:96–102.
51. Kamm MA, Dudding TC, Melenhorst J, et al. Sacral nerve stimulation for intractable constipation. Gut 2010;59:333–40.

Managing the Forgetful Patient

Best Practice for Cognitive Impairment

Catherine Nicastri, MD, Jennifer Hensley, MD, Susan Lane, MD*

KEYWORDS

- Cognitive impairment • Primary care • Dementia

KEY POINTS

- Primary care physicians are the frontline providers of patients with cognitive impairment.
- Perform yearly screening for cognitive impairment during the Medicare Annual Wellness Visit.
- Perform a thorough evaluation for diagnosis of dementia and exclude reversible causes when cognitive impairment is suspected.
- Refer to specialists when the diagnosis is uncertain and for assistance with therapeutics.
- Caring for patients with cognitive impairment requires a team approach and both non-pharmacological and pharmacologic treatments.

INTRODUCTION

The number of Americans living with dementia is increasing rapidly. In 2019, 5.8 million Americans were living with Alzheimer disease. Without new breakthroughs or treatments, Alzheimer disease is expected to affect 14 million Americans by 2050. Currently 1 in 10 seniors aged 65 years and older are living with dementia. Alzheimer disease is the sixth leading cause of death in the United States.

Results of a recent consumer survey demonstrated that although 94% of seniors had seen their primary care physician (PCP) for routine examinations in the past year, fewer than half had ever discussed memory concerns with their PCP. Although most of the seniors (82%) believe that having their memory evaluated is important, only 16% of seniors receive cognitive assessments.[1] PCPs are well positioned to provide front-line care for memory assessment. The Medicare Annual Wellness Visit (AWV) is an invaluable opportunity for early detection of cognitive decline in the primary care setting.

Department of Medicine, Renaissance School of Medicine at SUNY Stony Brook, Stony Brook University Hospital, HSC-T-16-020, 101 Nicolls Road, Stony Brook, NY 11794, USA
* Corresponding author.
E-mail address: Susan.Lane@stonybrookmedicine.edu

Med Clin N Am 105 (2021) 75–91
https://doi.org/10.1016/j.mcna.2020.09.001
0025-7125/21/© 2020 Elsevier Inc. All rights reserved.

NATURE OF THE PROBLEM

One of the earliest signs of dementia may be increasingly frequent or worsening episodes of confusion or memory loss. Most patients with dementia do not present with a self-complaint of memory loss; more often a spouse or another family member raises the concern. The personal experience of self-perceived worsening of cognitive function has been called subjective cognitive decline. Researchers have begun to focus on the importance of older adults reporting their memory and cognitive problems before a formal physician evaluation. Using the Behavioral Risk Factor Surveillance System survey, which includes questions on self-perceived confusion and memory loss, researchers found that although 11% of Americans aged 45 years and older reported subjective cognitive decline, more than half of those reporting this had not consulted a health care professional.[2] Subjective cognitive decline is an early warning sign of Alzheimer disease and may help to identify people at increased risk of developing dementia. Therefore, it is important for people experiencing memory loss to seek medical help to determine if the changes are normal, reversible, or a symptom of dementia.

Although forgetfulness is the most common presenting complaint in patients with dementia, difficulty with one or more of the following may also be present (**Box 1**).

DIAGNOSTIC CRITERIA

The Diagnostic and Statistical Manual of Mental Disorders Fifth edition (DSM-5) updated the diagnostic criteria of both dementia and mild cognitive impairment (CI), renaming them as major and minor neurocognitive disorders. Although memory decline may be seen with normal aging, function is not affected. Minor neurocognitive disorder is self-reported moderate cognitive decline that does not interfere with instrumental activities of daily living (IADLs). Major neurocognitive disorder requires demonstration of significant cognitive decline in one of the following domains—complex attention, executive function, language, learning and memory, perceptual motor or social cognition—and must interfere with IADLs[3] (**Table 1**).

| Box 1 |
| Ten early signs and symptoms of Alzheimer disease |

1. Memory loss that disrupts daily life
2. Challenges in planning or solving problems
3. Difficulty completing familiar tasks
4. Confusion with time or place
5. Trouble understanding visual images and special relationships
6. New problem with words in speaking or writing
7. Misplacing things and losing the ability to retrace steps
8. Decreased or poor judgment
9. Withdrawal from work or social activities
10. Changes in mood and personality

From 10 early Signs and Symptoms of Alzheimers. Alzheimer Association. https://www.alz.org/alzheimers-dementia/10_signs. Accessed May 10, 2020; with permission.

Table 1	
Diagnostic criteria for neurocognitive disorders	
Major Neurocognitive Disorder	**Minor Neurocognitive Disorder**
Evidence of significant cognitive decline from a previous level of performance in one or more cognitive domains • Complex attention • Executive function • Learning and memory • Language • Perceptual motor • Social cognition Based on: 1. Concern of the individual, a knowledgeable informant, or the clinician that there has been a significant decline in cognitive function; and 2. Substantial impairment in cognitive performance by neuropsychological testing (preferred) or another quantified clinical assessment.	Evidence of modest cognitive decline from a previous level of performance in one or more cognitive domains • Complex attention • Executive function • Learning and memory • Language • Perceptual motor • Social cognition Based on: 1. Concern of the individual, a knowledgeable informant, or the clinician that there has been a mild decline in cognitive function; and 2. Modest impairment in cognitive performance by neuropsychological testing (preferred) or another quantified clinical assessment.
The cognitive deficits interfere with IADLs	The cognitive deficits do not interfere with IADLS but may require greater effort or compensatory strategies
For both major and minor neurocognitive disorder diagnosis: • Cognitive deficits do not occur exclusively in the context of delirium • Cognitive deficits are not explained by another mental disorder (eg, depression)	
Specify whether due to • Alzheimer disease • Frontotemporal lobe degeneration • LBD • Vascular disease • Traumatic brain injury • Substance/medication use • HIV infection • Prion disease • PD • Huntington disease • Another medical condition • Multiple causes • Unspecified	

Abbreviation: HIV, human immunodeficiency virus.

Adapted from Neurocognitive Disorders. American Psychiatric Association: Diagnostic and Statistical Manual of Mental Disorders. 5th Ed. Arlington, VA: American Psychiatric Association; 2013; with permission.

TYPES OF DEMENTIA
Alzheimer Disease

Alzheimer disease is the most common cause of dementia accounting for 70% to 80% of cases. Alzheimer disease is characterized by the gradual onset of memory loss with language and visual impairments. Early signs include difficulty remembering recent names, events, or conversations and may be accompanied by apathy and depression.

Later symptoms include behavioral changes, disorientation, confusion, poor judgment, and impaired communication. Progression ultimately results in difficulty speaking, swallowing, and walking.[1]

Cerebrovascular Disease (Vascular Dementia)

Vascular dementia is the second most common cause of dementia accounting for up to 10% of cases and is typically described as a sudden or stepwise progression of memory deficits. Cognitive difficulties may be mild initially and gradually worsen as a result of multiple minor strokes or other conditions that affect smaller blood vessels of the brain leading to widespread damage. Vascular dementia often presents with impaired executive functioning including impaired ability to plan or organize, poor judgment, or impaired ability to make decisions. Difficulty with motor function such as slow gait and worsening balance may be seen.[1]

Lewy Body disease

Lewy body disease (LBD) is the third most common cause of memory loss affecting 5% to 10% of dementia patients. It is gradual in onset with symptoms overlapping with Alzheimer disease. Patients with LBD are more likely to have early symptoms of sleep disturbance, visual hallucinations, and parkinsonian movement features (eg, resting tremor, slowness and gait imbalance). Unlike Parkinson disease (PD), memory deficits tend to precede the parkinsonian features.[1]

Parkinson Disease

PD is a common, slowly progressive neurologic disorder affecting 2% of people older than 65 years. It often presents with motor slowness, rigidity, tremor, and changes in gait. Unlike LBD, the symptoms of movement disorder in PD proceed the memory deficits, with the average time to onset of dementia estimated at 10 years. Affected cognitive functions include short-term memory, attention, judgment, and understanding steps for task completion.[1]

Frontotemporal Lobe Degeneration

Frontotemporal disorders resulting from damage to neurons in the frontal and temporal lobe generally affect personality, behavior, language, and movement. Frontotemporal lobe degenerations (FTLDs) include behavior variant FTLD, primary progressive aphasia (PPA), corticobasal degeneration, and progressive supranuclear palsy (PSP). Approximately 60% of affected individuals are 45 to 64 years old. Although progressive, in the early stages, affected individuals may have just one symptom with short-term memory typically intact. In behavioral variant FTLD people may act strangely in social situations, may seem to lack empathy, and may not recognize their unusual behavior. Patients with primary progressive aphasia may have difficulty speaking or reading; however, their reasoning and judgment are not initially affected.[1]

Mixed Dementia

Individuals who show symptoms of more than one type of dementia such as Alzheimer and vascular disease are considered to have mixed pathologies, which may be more common than previously recognized. One study of people with dementia at Alzheimer disease centers showed that 50% had pathologic evidence of more than one cause of dementia.[4]

SCREENING FOR DEMENTIA

The United States Preventative Task Force has concluded there is insufficient evidence to recommend for or against routine screening for dementia in older adults. Despite this, the Centers for Medicare and Medicaid Service (CMS), through their AWV, requires detection of CI. The AWV benefit is largely underutilized, with only 19% of the 55.3 million eligible undergoing AWV.[5] CMS does not recommend a specific tool for the detection of CI, and currently there is no nationally recognized screening tool. In 2013 the Alzheimer's Association published its expert recommendation to incorporate cognitive assessment into the AWV and created a cognitive assessment toolkit (https://www.alz.org/media/documents/cognitive-assessment-toolkit.pdf).[6] The toolkit contains a Medicare AWV algorithm for assessment of cognition, validated patient, and informant assessment tools. The patient assessment tools are equal or superior to the Mini-Mental State Exam for detecting dementia, have been validated in the primary care setting, and can be administered by trained medical staff. Although there is no "one-size-fits-all" test for cognitive screening, there are numerous cognitive assessment tests, each with its own sensitivity, specificity, strengths, and limitations. Clinicians should determine which test is most appropriate for their practice, taking into consideration administration time and the patient's education level and level of impairment. See **Table 2** for comparison of common cognitive screening tests.

DIAGNOSIS AND EVALUATION OF DEMENTIA

Reversible causes of memory impairment should be ruled out with a thorough history including medication review, physical examination, laboratory testing, and neuroimaging. Evaluation includes assessment for metabolic derangements, thyroid function, depression, vitamin deficiencies, infectious causes, mass lesions, normal pressure hydrocephalus (NPH), vascular (ischemic vs vasculitis), or other neurologic causes of CI. See **Table 5** for a detailed list of reversible causes of dementia that should be excluded as part of the diagnostic evaluation.

HISTORY

A thorough history helps determine appropriate testing to limit unnecessary burden on the patient and family. Take a detailed history, including a safety history (**Box 2**), from the patient and a reliable informant to determine whether the symptoms are due to normal aging or mild or moderate neurocognitive disorder. The informant should know the patient's past and current levels of functioning including ADLs, IADLs, and executive functioning (**Table 3**).

Obtaining the history from the informant independently of the patient ensures reliable information that may not be obtainable with the patient present. The clinician should remain cognizant of cultural or religious beliefs, health literacy, and language barriers that may limit accuracy of the history.[15] Obtain permission to speak with others when the patient has capacity. When the patient is accompanied by a family member or caregiver, ensure that all participants feel included in the discussion through eye contact and by directly addressing each participant. When the patient with memory problems is unable to answer questions accurately, it is important to continue to engage them in the conversation. Be aware of cues from the companion as to the accuracy of answers as they may not want to contradict the patient. Arrange a time to gather more information privately, as the companion may have additional information to help you better care for your patient.

Table 2
Cognitive screening tests

Test	Components	Time to Administer (min)	Comments	Sensitivity (Sen) & Specificity (Spe)
General Practitioner Assessment of Cognition (GPCOG)[7,8] http://gpcog.com.au	Patient screen and informant screen	4 2	Validated in primary care setting No significant education bias Available in multiple languages Free	85% Sen 87% Spe
Mini-Cog (http://mini-cog.com)[9]	3-item recall and clock drawing	3	No education or language bias Available in multiple languages Free	76% Sen 73% Spe
Memory Impairment Screen (MIS)[10]	4-item delayed free and cued recall	4	Does not require ability to write Performance minimally affected by education level Available in multiple languages Cannot be used in people who are unable to read or who have visual impairment	79% Sen 91% Spe
Short Form of the Informant Questionnaire on Cognitive Decline in the Elderly (Short IQCOD)[10] https://www.alz.org/careplanning/downloads/cms-consensus.pdf	16-item informant-based questionnaire completed by relative/friend who has known patient >10 y	10–15	Validated in multiple languages Unaffected by education, premorbid ability, or language Results can be affected by mental health of informant and quality of relationship between informant and patient	Sen 89% Spe 82%
Ascertain Dementia 8-item Informant Questionnaire (AD8)[11,12]	8-item informant-based questionnaire	3	Validated in multiple languages Discriminates between normal aging and mild dementia May be completed before visit Can capture cognitive changes in high-functioning individuals, which may be missed on other screens	Sen 84% Spe 80%

| Montreal Cognitive Assessment (MoCA)[13,14] http://mocatest.org | 30-question test Measures executive function and multiple cognitive domains not measured by MMSE | 10 | Available in more than 200 languages Alternate versions to decrease learning effect from repeat testing Adapted for persons with physical and mental disabilities Will require certification to access tests after 9/1/2020 | 90% Sens 100% Spe With cut-off score of 26 for MCI |

Data from Refs.[7–14]

Box 2
Safety assessment question topics

- Driving
- Wandering
- Fires/oven and kitchen safety
- Falls
- Financial mismanagement
- Medication adherence
- Substance abuse
- Signs of neglect or abuse
- Home safety and supervision

It is important to diagnose and treat depression and anxiety disorders, as they may cause decreased attention, memory, and function and reduced quality of life.[16,17] **Table 4** lists several validated office-based screening tests to detect depression and anxiety in the elderly. Although validated in the geriatric population, the degree of CI may affect the tests' sensitivity and specificity. Referral to a geriatric psychiatrist and/or a neuropsychologist is necessary when the psychiatric diagnosis is unclear or when the patient is not responding to treatment.

MEDICATION REVIEW

Review medications that can contribute to CI, including over-the-counter medications and supplements, and verify that medications are taken as prescribed. Review all medications to determine their necessity and simplify the medication schedule to aid in adherence and ensure safety. The 2019 American Geriatrics Society Updated Beers Criteria for Potentially Inappropriate Medication Use in Older Adults includes medications that should be used with caution in the elderly; the risks of potential side effects or adverse reactions of these medications may outweigh the benefits in the absence of an alternative.[23] Any medications that may be contributing to worsening cognition should be discontinued with full consideration of withdrawal effects and worsening of other medical conditions. A helpful online resource for deprescribing can be found at https://deprescribing.org/. Assess whether the risk of an untreated

---

Table 3
Functional assessment

ADLS: Activity of Daily Living	IADLS: Instrumental	Executive
Dressing oneself	Shopping	Holding a job
Feeding oneself	Housekeeping	Organizing ability
Ambulating	Accounting	Multitasking
Able to toilet	Preparing meals	Computer skills
Hygiene and cleaning self	Medication management	Abstract concepts
Transferring	Telephoning	Planning and initiating tasks
	Arranging transportation	

Table 4	
Screening tests for psychiatric disorders	
Screening Tests	**Cause to Consider**
Patient Health Questionnaire-9 (PHQ-9)[18]	Depression
Patient Health Questionnaire-2 (PHQ-2)[18]	Depression
Geriatric Depression Scale (GDS)[19]	Depression
General Anxiety Disorder 7-item scale (GAD-7)[20]	Anxiety disorder
Short Anxiety Screening Test (SAST)[21]	Anxiety disorder
Patient Health Questionnaire-4 (PHQ-4)[22]	Depression and anxiety disorder

Data from Refs.[18–22]

condition or abruptly discontinuing one of these medications might cause more harm than the possibility of worsening cognition.[24]

Involving family or caregiver, pharmacist or a nursing agency in the care plan can improve medication safety. The National Institutes of Aging has an online resource available at https://www.nia.nih.gov/health/safe-use-medicines-older-adults that can help patients and family with adherence strategies. Some pharmacies provide individualized pill or blister packs, and home care nursing agencies can help with medication arrangements or educate the family about medication management.

PHYSICAL EXAMINATION

Perform a comprehensive physical examination to identify signs of neurologic, physical, or acute medical issues that could be contributing to memory loss. Notable examination findings (and their possible etiologies) include abnormal gait (PD, PSP), tremor and rigidity (PD), abnormal gaze (PSP, LBD), aphasia (PPA), and apraxia (early stage Alzheimer disease, late stage FTLD). The examination can guide further workup including cardiac testing, laboratory and microbiology testing, and neuroimaging.

LABORATORY TESTING

The American Academy of Neurology recommends routine blood work to screen for reversible causes of dementia (**Table 5**). These tests may not reveal a reversible cause of CI but can identify concomitant conditions that may exacerbate memory loss. Standard laboratories include complete blood count, metabolic panel, TSH, B12 level, and testing for infectious etiologies if there is concern for acute causes of memory loss such as delirium.[25,26] For example, because Lyme disease can cause neurologic manifestations such as CI, patients in endemic areas should be screened due to its reversibility with early treatment.[27]

NEUROIMAGING

Perform brain imaging on patients undergoing a workup for CI based on guidelines from The Alzheimer's Association International Conference 2018 and the American Academy of Neurology. Brain computed tomography (CT) can be done initially if there is concern for an acute bleed, subdural hematoma, or thrombotic stroke or if the patient will not tolerate or has a contraindication to MRI. Both CT and MRI can identify vascular disease and NPH. MRI and magnetic resonance angiography with and without contrast are more sensitive and should be performed when the

Table 5
Recommended laboratory testing

Laboratory or Imaging Test	Reversible Cause
TSH	Hypothyroidism
B12	Vitamin deficiency
Basic metabolic panel	Metabolic: hypercalcemia, hyponatremia, uncontrolled diabetes, renal failure
CBC	Anemia
Liver function	Hepatic encephalopathy
Urinalysis & culture	Urinary tract infection
ESR	Nonspecific for inflammation, infection, malignancy
Infectious disease (when indicated by history): HIV RPR Lyme ELISA with reflex to western blot	AIDS dementia Tertiary syphilis Lyme disease

Abbreviations: CBC, complete blood count; ELISA, enzyme-linked immunosorbent assay; ESR, erythrocyte sedimentation rate; HIV, human immunodeficiency virus; RPR, rapid plasma regain test; TSH, thyroid stimulating hormone.

patient has atypical symptoms such as early onset (age <65 years), rapid decline or sudden symptoms, or other focal neurologic findings (weakness, tremor, rigidity, gait, and balance difficulties) to rule out mass lesions, multiple sclerosis, vasculitis, or infection.[26,28,29]

Neuropsychological testing is useful in patients who complain of memory deficits or a change in executive function who have higher education and/or intelligence or who perform well on screening tests. Neuropsychological testing also helps to monitor progression of cognitive impairment.

Refer to a neurologist or dementia specialist when the diagnosis is uncertain, when atypical symptoms are present (hallucinations, personality changes, disinhibition), when neurologic changes are observed (gait disturbance, postural instability), in the setting of rapidly progressive cognitive decline, or in a younger patient (<65 years) exhibiting early onset memory loss. Refer to a geriatric psychiatrist when there are behavior symptoms that pose a threat to patient or caregiver safety or when the patient is not responding to treatment. Social workers and adult protective services can help with psychosocial issues including concerns of abuse, safety, and hardship.

TREATMENT AND MANAGEMENT

Once the diagnosis of dementia is made, both nonpharmacological and pharmacologic care should begin. At every visit, the PCP should assess safety as well as cognitive and functional decline (see **Box 2**, **Tables 2** and **3**). If there is an acute or rapid decline in function and/or cognition, determine whether there is a reversible cause other than dementia progression to explain the decline. Functional assessment helps the physician identify the stage of dementia (**Table 6**), which directs when to start and discontinue medications and the overall plan for goals of care. The Global Deterioration Scale or Reisberg Scale was developed to depict the stages of the most common

Table 6		
Stages of dementia (The Global Deterioration Scale/Reisberg Scale)		
Diagnosis	**Stage**	**Signs and Symptoms**
No dementia	Stage 1: No cognitive decline	Normal functioning without memory loss
No dementia	Stage 2: Very mild cognitive decline	Normal forgetfulness with aging
No dementia	Stage 3: Mild cognitive decline	Increasing forgetfulness, some difficulty with concentrating and work performance. Maybe noticed by family.
Early-stage	Stage 4: Moderate cognitive decline *Mild dementia*	Worsening difficulty with concentration, recent memories, and difficulty managing finances or traveling alone to new locations. Trouble completing complex tasks. Denial of symptoms but deficiencies can be detected by the physician.
Mid-stage	Stage 5: Moderately severe cognitive decline *Moderate dementia*	Major memory deficiencies such as not oriented to the date, time, location, residence. Patient may need some assistance with ADLs.
Mid-stage	Stage 6: Severe cognitive decline (middle dementia) *Moderately severe dementia*	Needs assistance to complete ADLs and finish tasks. Complete assistance with hygiene and toileting. Unable to remember close family members' names or relationships. Unable to recall recent events such as last meal. Forgets major past events such as death of parents. May have delusions, agitation, anxiety, and hallucinations.
Late-stage	Stage 7: Very severe cognitive decline (late dementia) *Severe dementia*	Minimally verbal or unable to communicate. Require assistance with all ADLs. At end of this stage, they are bedbound and unable to ambulate or move on their own. Qualify for hospice care.

(*Revised from* https://www.dementiacarecentral.com/aboutdementia/facts/stages/#scales 33; with permission.)[30,31]

form of dementia, Alzheimer disease; symptoms can vary at each stage with the different types of dementia.

THE TEAM APPROACH TO CARE

Dementia is typically a progressive disease that requires a team-based approach. Maintain a patient-centered approach, with each team member contributing to the care plan and working to ensure safety and respect for the patient's goals of care. The members of the team and their roles include the following:

Patient: tailor the plan to best fit the needs of the individual patient based on the patient's beliefs, values, and expressed goals of care.

Caregiver: the caregiver may be a member of the family, a spouse, a paid aide, or a friend. Assess the caregiver's role and determine the individual's level of commitment, responsibility, and reliability. Assess the caregiver's needs, as they often have stressors that are overlooked, which may affect patient care. Consider the caregiver's health literacy level when reviewing the plan of care.

Social worker (SW): early referral to SW is vital to assess the support system for later stages. The SW can assess home safety and the relationships of support among family and friends. The SW can identify community support services available such as Meals on Wheels, transportation services, day programs, local charity services, and home health aide agencies and can assist with Medicaid applications and insurance.

Home care agencies: nursing agencies can perform home safety assessments, medication reconciliation and management, help manage comorbid conditions, and educate the patient and family. A nursing agency can arrange in-home physical and occupational therapy, speech pathology, and SW services. Nursing can complete a Patient Review Instrument to assess appropriateness for nursing home care.

Clinic nursing and support staff: coordination of the care plan includes transitional care visits, phone calls to review medication changes, and changes in care needs postdischarge from the hospital. Staff can assist with medication reconciliation, coordinating appointments, testing, and referrals to consultants.

PCP: coordinates care with the team while managing patient symptoms, comorbidities, and medications. Advanced care planning discussions, including health care proxy designation, should occur early in the diagnosis to allow the patient to maintain autonomy and define personal preferences and goals of care. The Medical Orders for Life Sustaining Treatment (https://molst.org/) and the Physician Orders for Life Sustaining Treatment (https://polst.org/) are forms that the PCP can use to initiate these discussions.

Elder care attorney: an elder care attorney can assist with advance care planning including Last Will and Testament, Living Will, Health Care Proxy, and Power of Attorney designations.

NONPHARMACOLOGIC THERAPY FOR MANAGEMENT OF DEMENTIA

Treatment of dementia should target cognitive and functional decline. Nonpharmacologic therapies focus on improving cognition and function and reducing neuropsychiatric symptoms such as agitation, anxiety, irritability, delusions, and sleep changes.

COGNITIVE THERAPY

In the early stages of dementia, cognitive training and rehabilitation helps patients to maintain memory and executive functioning and to devise strategies to compensate for declining function. Cognitive training focuses on identifying and addressing an individual's needs and goals and developing strategies to take in new information using compensatory methods such as memory aides.[32]

EXERCISE

Structured exercise programs may improve the ability to perform ADLs in people with mild to severe dementia. Exercise should be recommended because slowing the progression of ADL dependence has significant benefit for families and caregivers and the patient's quality of life; it may also delay the need for long-term care placement.[33]

Table 7
Food and Drug Administration approved medications

Class	Medication	Indications	Common Side Effects	Precautions
Cholinesterase inhibitors (CI)	Donepezil	Mild, moderate, and severe AD	All CI: nausea, vomiting, diarrhea, abdominal pain, anorexia	All CI: QT prolongation, bradycardia; use with caution with LBBB, SSS, AV nodal block
	Rivastigmine	Mild, moderate AD and Parkinson-related dementia TD patch: mild, moderate, and severe AD and mild to moderate PD	Muscle cramps Headache and dizziness, tremor, skin rash Patch has fewer GI side effects	Use with caution: urinary retention gastric ulcer disease Asthma/COPD
	Galantamine	Mild to moderate AD	Dizziness	
N-methyl-ᴅ-aspartate (NMDA) receptor antagonist	Memantine	Moderate to severe AD	Confusion and drowsiness; Less common: dizziness, headaches, constipation, hypertension, and hallucinations	Use with caution in cardiovascular disease, hepatic impairment, seizures, severe renal and ophthalmic disease

Abbreviations: AD, Alzheimer disease; AV, atrioventricular block; COPD, chronic obstructive pulmonary disease; LBBB, left bunble branch block; SSS, sick sinus syndrome; TD, transdermal.
Data from Refs.[37,38].

OCCUPATIONAL THERAPY

Occupational therapy to train patients and their caregivers' techniques for coping with CI has been shown to improve motor and process skills and ADLs. Individualized therapy sessions should focus on training patient and caregiver on the use of aides as well as teaching coping behaviors and strategies to compensate for functional deficits.[34]

NONPHARMACOLOGIC BEHAVIORAL MANAGEMENT

Behavioral and psychological symptoms of dementia such as apathy, depression, irritability, agitation, anxiety, disinhibition, delusions, hallucinations, delusions, and sleep changes are highly prevalent and are some of the most distressing symptoms of dementia for patients and caregivers.[35] It is beneficial to identify triggers that exacerbate behavioral and psychological symptoms and to implement nonpharmacological practices (eg, massage, multisensory stimulation, reminiscence therapy, music and pet therapy) that are person centered, evidence based, and feasible in the care setting.[36]

PHARMACOLOGIC THERAPY

There are 4 Food and Drug Administration-approved drugs for dementia from 2 medication classes: acetylcholinesterase inhibitors and N-methyl-D-aspartate agonists (**Table 7**). The medications do not halt the progression of dementia but may delay the decline within various cognitive and functional domains. Start with the lowest dose and titrate up over time to improve tolerability; refer to dosing from a reputable source or hospital formulary.

SUMMARY

The optimal care of the forgetful patient in the primary care office involves a team approach to ensure safety and to improve the quality of life for the patient and caregiver. The initial workup and diagnosis of memory loss includes a thorough history, medication review, physical examination, laboratory testing, and appropriate imaging. The PCP must monitor the patient as the disease progresses to determine the resources required to ensure that the patient's needs are met. Treatment should focus on pharmacologic and nonpharmacological therapy.

CLINICS CARE POINTS

- Most seniors believe having their memory evaluated is important but only 16% receive cognitive assessments.
- In patients with suspected dementia validated screening tools such as the mini-cog, GPCOG, AD8 should be performed to determine need for further evaluation.
- Reversible causes of memory impairment should be ruled out with a thorough history including medication review, physical examination, laboratory testing, and neuroimaging.
- People with dementia should have a structured assessment before starting nonpharmacological or pharmacological treatment for memory or behavioral problems.
- Treatment with both nonpharmacological and pharmacologic care should be initiated once the diagnosis of dementia is made.

- Referral to specialists such as neuropsychologist, neurologist or geriatric psychiatrist is valuable for help with less common disorders and complicated psychological or behavioral changes.

DISCLOSURE

The authors have nothing to disclose.

REFERENCES

1. Alzheimer's Association. 2019 Alzheimer's Disease Facts and Figures. Alzheimers Dement 2019;15(3):321–87.
2. Taylor CA, Bouldin ED, McGuire LC. Subjective cognitive decline among adults aged >45 years. MMWR Morb Mortal Wkly Rep 2018;67(27):753–7.
3. Neurocognitive disorders. American psychiatric Association: diagnostic and Statistical Manual of Mental disorders. 5th edition. Arlington (VA): American Psychiatric Association; 2013.
4. Brenowitz WD, Hubbard RA, Keene CD, et al. Mixed neuropathologies and estimated rates of clinical progression in a large autopsy sample. Alzheimers Dement 2017;13(6):654–62.
5. Cordell CB, Malaz B, Joshua C, et al. ALzheimer's Association recommendations for operationalizing the detection of cognitive impairment during the Medicare Annual Wellness Visit in a primary care setting. Alzheimers Dement 2013;9: 141–50.
6. Cognitive Assessment Toolkit. Alzheimer Association. Available at: https://www.alz.org/media/documents/cognitive-assessment-toolkit.pdf. Accessed May 10, 2020.
7. Brodaty H, Pond D, Kep NM, et al. The GPCOG: a new screening test for dementia designed for general practice. J Am Geriatr Soc 2002;50(3):530–4.
8. Brodaty H, Connors MH, Loy C, et al. Screening for Dementia in Primary Care: A comparison of the GPCOG and the MMSE. Dement Geriatr Cogn Disord 2016; 42(5–6):323–30.
9. Holsinger T, Plassman BL, Stechuchak KM, et al. Screening for cognitive impairment: comparing the performance of four instruments in primary care. J Am Geriatr Soc 2012;60(6):1027–36.
10. Tsoi KK, Chan JY, Hirai HW, et al. Cognitive tests to detect dementia: a systematic review and meta-analysis. JAMA Intern Med 2015;175(9):1450–8.
11. Galvin JE, Roe CM, Powlishta KK, et al. The AD8: A brief informant interview to detect dementia. Neurology 2005;65(4):559–64.
12. Galvin JE, Roe CM, Xiong C, et al. Validity and Reliability of the AD8 informant interview in dementia. Neurology 2006;67(11):1942–8.
13. Nasreddine ZS, Phillips NA, Bedirian V, et al. The Montreal Cognitive Assessment, MoCA: a brief screening tool for mild cognitive impairment. J Am Geriatr Soc 2005;53(4):695–9.
14. MoCA Montreal Cognitive Asessment. Available at: https://www.mocatest.org/. Accessed May 1, 2020.
15. Shaji KS, Sivakumar PT, Prasad Rao GP, et al. Clinical practice guidelines for management of dementia. Indian J Psychiatry 2018;60(3):312–28.
16. Perini G, Ramusino MC, Sinforiani E, et al. Cognitive impairment in depression: recent advances and novel treatments. Neuropsychiatr Dis Treat 2019;15: 1249–58.

17. Beaudreau SA, O'Hara R. Late-life anxiety and cognitive impairment: a review. Am J Geriatr Psychiatry 2008;16(10):790–803.

18. Boyle LL, Richardson TM, He H, et al. How do the phq-2, the phq-9 perform in aging services clients with cognitive impairment? Int J Geriatr Psychiatry 2011; 26(9):952–60.

19. Conradsson M, Rosendahl E, Littbrand H, et al. Usefulness of the Geriatric Depression Scale 15-item version among very old people with and without cognitive impairment. Aging Ment Health 2013;17(5):638–45.

20. Spitzer RL, Kroenke KM, Williams JB, et al. A brief measure for assessing Generalized Anxiety Disorder: the GAD-7. Arch Intern Med 2006;166(10):1092–7.

21. Sinoff G, Ore L, Zlotogorsky D, et al. Short Anxiety Screening Test–a brief instrument for detecting anxiety in the elderly. Int J Geriatr Psychiatry 1999;14(12): 1062–71.

22. Kroenke K, Spitzer RL, Williams JB, et al. An Ultra-Brief Screening Scale for Anxiety and Depression: The PHQ–4. Psychosomatics 2009;50(6):613–21.

23. The 2019 American Geriatrics Society Beers Criteria Expert Panel. American Geriatrics Society 2019 Updated AGS Beers Criteria for Potentially Inappropriate Medication Use in Older Adults. J Am Geriatr Soc 2019;67(4):674–94.

24. Lisi DM. Definition of Drug-Induced Cognitive Impairment in the Elderly. Medscape Pharmacotherapy. 2000. Available at: https://www.medscape.com/viewarticle/408593_5. Accessed May 1, 2020.

25. Weytingh MD, Bossuyt PMM, van Crevel H. Reversible Dementia: more than 10% or less than 1%? A quantitative review. J Neurol 1995;242(7):466–71.

26. Knopman DS, DeKosky ST, Cummings JL, et al. Practice parameter: Diagnosis of Dementia (an evidence-based review) Report of the Quality Standards Subcommittee of the American Academy of Neurology. Neurology 2001;56(9):1143–53.

27. Blanc F, Philippi N, Cretin B, et al. Lyme neuroborreliosis and dementia. J Alzheimers Dis 2014;41(4):1087–93.

28. Alzheimer's Association Workgroup. From the alzheimer's association international conference 2018: first practice guidelines for clinical evaluation of alzheimer's disease and other dementias for primary and specialty care. 2018. Available at: https://www.alz.org/aaic/downloads2018/Sun-clinical-practice-guidelines.pdf. Accessed May 5, 2020.

29. Darrow MD. A practical approach to dementia in the outpatient primary care setting. Prim Care 2015;42:195–204.

30. Reisberg B, Ferris SH, de Leon MJ, et al. The global deterioration scale for assessment of primary degenerative dementia. Am J Psychiatry 1982;139: 1136–9.

31. Morris JC. The Clinical dementia treating (CDR): Current version and scoring rules. Neurology 1993;43:2412.

32. Bahar-Fuchs A, Martyr A, Goh AM, et al. Cognitive training for people with mild to moderate dementia. Cochrane Database Syst Rev 2019;25(3):CD013069.

33. Forbes D, Forbes SC, Blake CM, et al. Exercise programs for people with dementia. Cochrane Database Syst Rev 2015;15(4):CD006489.

34. Graff MJ, Vernooij-Dasseh MJ, Thijssen M, et al. Community Based Occupational Therapy for Patients with Dementia and their Care-givers: randomised control trial. BMJ 2006;333:1196–9.

35. Steinberg M, Shao H, Zandi P, et al. Point and 5-year period prevalence of neuropsychiatric symptoms in dementia: The Cache County study. Int J Geriatr Psychiatry 2008;23(2):170–7.

36. Scales K, Zimmerman S, Miller S. Evidence-Based Nonpharmacological Practices to Address Behavioral and Psychological Symptoms of Dementia. Gerontologist 2018;58(S1):S88–102.
37. Rodda J, Carter J. Cholinesterase inhibitors and memantine for symptomatic treatment of dementia. BMJ 2012;344(7856):43–7.
38. Qaseem A, Snow V, Cross JT Jr, et al. Current pharmacologic treatment of dementia: a clinical practice guideline from the American College of Physicians and the American Academy of Family Physicians. Ann Intern Med 2008;148(5): 370–8.

Evidence-Based Approach to Palpitations

Clara Weinstock, DO*, Hilary Wagner, DO, Meghan Snuckel, MD, Marilyn Katz, MD

KEYWORDS

- Palpitations • Workup • Diagnose • Ambulatory ECG • Primary care • Heart monitor

KEY POINTS

- All patients presenting with a chief complaint of palpitations should undergo a detailed history, physical examination, and electrocardiogram (ECG).
- A thorough history is key in helping to diagnose the cause of the palpitations and is important in triaging which patients will need additional evaluation.
- Physical examination is low yield for diagnosing the cause of palpitations but should be used to guide further workup.
- A 2-week continuous loop event monitor has the highest diagnostic yield to cost ratio and is the test of choice when pursuing ambulatory ECG monitoring. Holter monitors should play a limited role in the evaluation of palpitations and should only be used when the patient's typical symptoms reliably occur at least every 24 hours.
- Consumer grade wearable devices such as smartwatches have potential for medical use in the future, but current data show their accuracy to be variable and their likelihood of finding clinically irrelevant abnormalities to be high.

INTRODUCTION

Palpitations are a common chief complaint and can be seen in a variety of settings including primary care, urgent care, the emergency department, and cardiology offices. The complaint of palpitations can refer to tachycardia, skipped beats, premature beats, or fluttering in the chest. The prevalence of palpitations in the community is 6% to 11%.[1,2] In a study evaluating the prevalence of chief complaints from multiple outpatient primary care offices, 16% of patients indicated that palpitations were a "major problem" for them.[3] Palpitations are also the second most common reason for referral to cardiology.[4]

A retrospective cohort study compared 109 patients who presented to primary care with palpitations with age- and sex-matched controls who did not report palpitations over a 5-year period and found no difference in the incidence of morbidity

University of Connecticut School of Medicine, 263 Farmington Avenue, Outpatient Pavilion-2nd Floor East, Farmington, CT 06030, USA
* Corresponding author.
E-mail address: clweinstock@uchc.edu

Med Clin N Am 105 (2021) 93–106
https://doi.org/10.1016/j.mcna.2020.09.004
0025-7125/21/© 2020 Elsevier Inc. All rights reserved.

and mortality between these 2 groups.[5] The overall mortality rate of patients with palpitations in a study by Weber and Kapoor was also low at 1.6%. Although overall morbidity and mortality is low, they found that palpitations resulted in missed work days (12% of patients), self-reported decreased work productivity (19% of patients), and accomplishing less than usual amount of work at home (33% of patients).[6]

It is therefore important to pursue a cost-conscious, evidence-based approach to evaluation and workup of palpitations. This article outlines the evidence behind the history, physical examination, laboratories, electrocardiogram (ECG), and additional testing modalities for patients presenting to primary care with palpitations.

Differential Diagnosis of Palpitations

Any arrhythmia, including sinus tachycardia, atrial fibrillation, premature ventricular contractions, ventricular tachycardia, and myocardial infarction can cause palpitations. There are noncardiac reasons for palpitations as well, including anxiety, thyroid issues, medications etc. Hypertrophic obstructive cardiomyopathy (HOCM) and ventricular tachycardia represent a small proportion of patients presenting with palpitations but are red flag diagnoses that can lead to sudden cardiac death. **Box 1** displays a broader differential diagnosis for palpitations.

In the Weber and Kapoor study described earlier, the cause of palpitations was found to be cardiac in 43% of patients, psychiatric in 31%, other in 10%, and unknown in 16%. Forty percent of the causes could be determined with the history and physical examination, an ECG, and/or laboratory data.[6] **Table 1** displays the prevalence breakdown of the different causes of palpitations in this study.

PATIENT HISTORY
Importance of History

Palpitations are a nonspecific symptom; the differential diagnosis of their origin is broad. A detailed patient history can help narrow the scope of further testing.

History of Present Illness

When did the palpitations start? Did the palpitations start suddenly or gradually? One study showed that the longer the palpitation lasts, the more likely it is to be related to an arrhythmia rather than a noncardiac cause.[7] On the other hand, palpitations that last for only a moment are more likely to represent premature ventricular contractions (PVCs) or premature atrial contractions. Sustained palpitations, lasting for minutes (or longer), are more consistent with supraventricular arrhythmias, ventricular arrhythmias, or anxiety.[8]

Where was the patient when the palpitations began and what were they doing? Sitting at rest could be a sign of vagal nerve-mediated cause (eg, ventricular premature contraction), whereas occurring with exercise or exertion that could lead to dehydration suggests worsening of mitral valve prolapse cardiomyopathy or exertional syncope.[9] One study showed that palpitations that occurred at work or palpitations that awoke one from sleep were significantly more likely to have a cardiac cause.[7] Onset while speaking in front of a large group of people could suggest a more benign origin such as anxiety or supraventricular tachycardia. Posture and postural changes are also important to note. For instance, atrioventricular nodal reentrant tachycardias have been described as being triggered by standing up after bending over. Supraventricular tachycardia and ventricular premature contractions have often been noted while the patient is lying in bed.[10]

Box 1
Differential diagnosis of palpitations

Cardiac—Arrhythmia
  Atrial fibrillation/flutter
  Bradycardia caused by arteriovenous block or sinus node dysfunction
  Brugada syndrome
  Multifocal atrial tachycardia
  Premature supraventricular or ventricular contractions
  Sinus tachycardia or arrhythmia
  Supraventricular tachycardia
  Ventricular tachycardia
  Wolf-Parkinson-White syndrome/long QT syndrome
  Pacemaker-mediated tachycardia

Cardiac—Structure
  Atrial or ventricular septal defect
  Atrial myxoma
  Cardiomyopathy
  Congenital heart disease
  Congestive heart failure
  Valvular disease (mitral valve prolapse, aortic insufficiency, aortic stenosis)

Drugs, Medications, Toxins
  Alcohol
  Tobacco/nicotine
  Caffeine
  Street drugs (cocaine, amphetamines, anabolic steroids, marijuana, ecstasy, heroin)
  Prescription medications (beta agonists, theophylline, digitalis, phenothiazine, steroids,
  methylphenidate, midodrine, epinephrine, anticholinergics)
  Over-the-counter medications (pseudoephedrine, omega-3-polyunsaturated fatty acids,
  coenzyme Q10, carnitine)
  Withdrawal of medications (beta-blockers)

Physiologic
  Exercise
  Fever
  Hypovolemia/dehydration
  Pregnancy

Endocrinologic
  Hyperthyroidism
  Hypoglycemia
  Paget disease of the bone
  Pheochromocytoma

Hematologic
  Anemia
  Mastocytosis

Psychological
  Anxiety, stress
  Panic attacks

Neurologic
  Autonomic dysfunction
  Vasovagal syndrome
  Postural Orthostatic Tachycardia Syndrome

Other
  Electrolyte Imbalance
  Pulmonary Disease

Courtesy of A. Abbott, M.D., Los Angeles, California.

Table 1
Prevalence of causes of palpitations in Weber and Kapoor study

Causes of Palpitations	No.	Percent
Cardiac	82	43.2
Atrial fibrillation	19	10
Supraventricular tachycardia	18	9.5
Premature ventricular beats	15	7.9
Atrial flutter	11	5.8
Premature atrial beats	6	3.2
Ventricular tachycardia	4	2.1
Mitral valve prolapse	2	1.1
Sick sinus syndrome	2	1.1
Pacemaker failure	2	1.1
Aortic insufficiency	2	1.1
Atrial myxoma	1	0.5
Psychiatric	58	30.5
Panic attack or disorder plus anxiety	20	10.5
Panic attack alone	17	8.9
Panic disorder alone	14	7.4
Anxiety alone	6	3.2
Panic plus anxiety plus somatization	1	0.5
Miscellaneous	19	10
Medication	5	2.6
Thyrotoxicosis	5	2.6
Caffeine	3	1.6
Cocaine	2	1.1
Anemia	2	1.1
Amphetamine	1	0.5
Macrocytosis	1	0.5
Unknown	31	16.3

From Weber BE, Kapoor WN. Evaluation and outcomes of patients with palpitations. The American Journal of Medicine. 1996;14(6):138-148; with permission.

Ask your patient to carefully describe the quality of the palpitation. A feeling of rapid fluttering in the chest is typically seen in sustained ventricular or supraventricular arrhythmias, including sinus tachycardia. The regularity or irregularity of the palpitation may indicate what is causing the arrhythmia. As described by Zimetbaum and Josephson, a sensation of "flip-flopping" in the chest, the experience of a pounding, or very strong heart beat followed by the heart briefly "stopping" may be caused by premature supraventricular or ventricular beats.[8] An irregular, pounding feeling in the neck along with palpitations has been reported by patients with PVCs, complete heart block, pacemaker syndrome, or ventricular tachycardia.[11] Patients frequently describe a feeling of an "unpleasant awareness" with aortic regurgitation.[12] **Table 2** summarizes some typical palpitation descriptions and the diagnosis with which they are classically associated. Patients with palpitations on a regular basis were more than twice as likely to have a significant cardiac arrhythmia as a cause for their palpitations versus those who did not describe any regularity to their palpitations.[7]

Table 2
Key clinical findings with palpitations and suggested diagnoses

Finding	Suggested Diagnosis
Single skipped beats	Benign ectopy
Feeling of being unable to catch one's breath	Ventricular premature contractions
Single pounding sensations	Ventricular premature contractions
Rapid regular pounding in neck	Supraventricular arrhythmias
Palpitations since childhood	Supraventricular tachycardia
Palpitations terminated by vagal maneuvers	Supraventricular tachycardia
Palpitations that are worse at night	Benign ectopy or atrial fibrillation
Rapid irregular rhythm	Atrial fibrillation, tachycardia with variable block
Palpitations associated with emotional distress	Psychiatric cause or catecholamine-sensitive arrhythmia
General anxiety	Panic attacks
Palpitations associated with activity	Coronary heart disease
Rapid palpitations with exercise	Supraventricular arrhythmia, palpitations associated with exercise
Medication or recreational drug use	Drug-induced palpitations
Positional palpitations	Atrioventricular nodal tachycardia, pericarditis
Friction rub	Pericarditis
Heat intolerance, tremor, thyromegaly	Hyperthyroidism
Heart murmur	Heart valve disease
Midsystolic click	Mitral valve prolapse

The information in this table is based on clinical experience and not data from clinical trials.
Courtesy of A. Abbott, M.D., Los Angeles, California.

Symptoms associated with the noncardiac causes outlined in **Box 1** are important to investigate to help build a differential. For instance, palpitations associated with heat intolerance could be associated with hyperthyroidism, whereas fever may indicate infection. Shortness of breath or choking sensation, nausea, dizziness, chest pain/discomfort, and paresthesias may help guide the diagnosis toward anxiety or panic attack.

Past Medical History

Past medical history is equally important as anxiety is the most common noncardiac cause of palpitations.[11] One study showed that a patient's palpitations are more likely to be of psychiatric nature if the patient is young, has a disability, has shown hypochondria-like behavior, or has been previously diagnosed with a somatization disorder.[13] The prevalence of an underlying panic disorder in patients with palpitations is 15% to 31%.[6] If it is thought that anxiety is playing a role, a clinician could use the Generalized Anxiety Disorder 7 item scale (GAD-7), a validated assessment tool to further assess the severity of symptoms. Other associated symptoms, including impending doom, diaphoresis, perioral numbness, and peripheral numbness, can help point to a diagnosis of anxiety or panic attack. It is important to remember that a person experiencing anxiety may have an underlying structural or additional medical reason for the palpitations. One study showed that 13% of patients diagnosed with a psychiatric disorder had a nonpsychiatric cause of their palpitations,[13] so anxiety as the sole cause should remain a diagnosis of exclusion until after proper testing has been completed.

Medications

Many medications, whether prescription, over the counter, or herbal supplements, can trigger palpitations, so a complete medication reconciliation is paramount. Antidepressants and benzodiazepines have been shown to be associated with a decreased risk of cardiac arrhythmia, whereas the use of beta-blockers, diuretics, angiotensin-converting enzyme inhibitors, and other antihypertensives correlated with an increased risk of cardiac arrhythmia.[7] Changes in dose or withdrawal can also be a source of palpitations, so ask for recent changes in dosage or frequency of use. Over-the-counter medications such as nasal decongestants with pseudoephedrine, omega-3-polyunsaturated fatty acids, coenzyme Q10, and carnitine have all been shown to cause palpitations.[14]

Social History

Caffeine is a common culprit for palpitations and is integral in many patient's routines. Cigarettes and other nicotine products also can trigger palpitations. Although cocaine and methamphetamines are commonly associated with palpitations and a combination of both accounts for 1.6% of patients presenting with palpitations,[6] marijuana has additionally been shown to cause arrhythmias.[15] Athletes and weight lifters may have tried performance-enhancing drugs such as anabolic steroids.[15]

Family History

A family history of diseases such as those described in **Box 1** can also help direct workup for palpitations. Prolonged QT syndrome and cardiomyopathies can run in families, as well as anxiety and thyroid disease. Ask your patient specifically if anyone in their family passed away from or had a heart attack before the age of 55 years for men and 65 years for women.[16]

PHYSICAL EXAMINATION

The physical examination, although a wonderful tool, can have low yield for patients with palpitations. This is likely due to the intermittent nature of palpitations, resulting in lack of symptoms at the time of presentation to the office. However, it can be helpful in ruling out many causes and help to refine the differential diagnosis.

The general appearance of the patient is important for many cardiac causes, particularly that of a myocardial infarction. Apparent distress due to pain or shortness of breath will alter the urgency of the workup.

Reviewing vital signs, even if within the normal range, can be an important clue in the workup for palpitations, particularly a change from the individual's baseline. For instance, an increase in the heart rate and a decrease in weight may indicate an excess of thyroid hormone. Although lung causes are less commonly associated with palpitations, an increased heart rate or respiratory rate and low pulse oximetry may indicate a pulmonary-induced cause such as multifocal atrial tachycardia or a pulmonary embolus. A lower blood pressure or orthostatic hypotension may indicate volume depletion. Orthostatic vital signs can also diagnose postural orthostatic tachycardia syndrome (POTS), which usually presents with complaints of intermittent palpitations and lightheadedness or syncope. POTS is characterized as orthostatic tachycardia, with an increase in heart rate by greater than 30 bpm (or an increase to

≥120 bpm) when moving from lying down to standing position, in the absence of orthostatic hypotension.[17] If there is clinical suspicion of POTS, a set of orthostatic blood pressures with pulse can make the diagnosis.

If a patient is actively having palpitations, a simple pulse check can begin to narrow the differential greatly, especially for arrhythmia-induced palpitations. An irregular pulse would lead a practitioner to think of atrial fibrillation or premature ventricular contractions. A retrospective study by Zeldis and colleagues reviewed charts of 477 patients presenting with cardiovascular complaints including palpitations, dyspnea, chest pain, dizziness, or syncope who underwent one or more 24-hour ECG monitor recordings. Of those with an irregular pulse on examination, 91% had a significant arrhythmia on 24-hour ECG (positive predictive value of 91%) and of those with a regular pulse on examination, 28% had a significant arrhythmia on their 24-hour ECG.[18] The sensitivity of an irregular pulse for significant arrhythmia on ECG in this study was only 7%. Thus, you would not have an irregular pulse on examination in most patients with significant arrhythmia on 24-hour ECG, but if you do detect an irregular pulse on examination then there is a very high chance of also detecting a significant arrhythmia on ambulatory ECG monitoring. No other single history or physical examination finding in this study could reliably predict detecting a significant arrhythmia on ambulatory ECG monitoring.

Point of maximal impulse (PMI), which is determined by careful palpation of the chest wall to determine the location of the apex, can be useful in assessing cardiomegaly, particularly if it is displaced laterally and inferiorly. Noting the strength of the PMI is also useful as stronger or weaker than anticipated may indicate a cardiac cause of palpitations.

Heart auscultation is useful with structural heart causes. Mitral valve prolapse has the classic sound of a mid- to late systolic click, and can be seen in isolation, or in conjunction with hyperthyroidism, particularly in young white women.[19] Some other murmurs that are commonly associated with the symptom of palpitations include aortic regurgitation and diastolic tumor plop. Aortic regurgitation is described as a soft high-pitched early diastolic decrescendo murmur. Links to audio clips of these murmurs can be found in **Box 2**.

Examination findings that could point to a thyroid cause include exophthalmos and/or lid lag, thyromegaly and/or thyroid nodules, diaphoresis, hand tremor, hyperreflexia, widened pulse pressure, and irregular or elevated heart beat.

Although not as common of a presentation, anemia can also present with palpitations, therefore looking for evidence of anemia on examination is reasonable. Individuals with anemia may have diastolic flow murmur, pallor of the conjunctiva, nail beds, and/or oral mucosa, or splenomegaly. In a 2017 study, researchers looked at signs/symptoms of severe anemia (hemoglobin less than or equal to 7%) in 94 patients.

Box 2
Murmur sound clips

Mitral valve prolapse—Heart Sounds. Medzcool https://www.youtube.com/watch?v=sH_KmHIHR70. Accessed March 30, 2020.

Aortic Regurgitation—Heart Sounds.; 2019. https://www.youtube.com/watch?v=uZysrKXHJMM. Accessed March 30, 2020.

From Medzcool. Mitral Valve Prolapse - Heart Sounds. Youtube. Available at: https://www.youtube.com/watch?v=sH_KmHIHR70. Accessed March 30, 2020; and Medzcool. Aortic Regurgitation - Heart Sounds. Available at: https://www.youtube.com/watch?v=uZysrKXHJMM.

They found that 54 patients out of the 94 had a cardiac murmur and when followed-up, most of these patients' murmur resolved after treatment of their anemia. The same study showed that 39 out of the 94 (41%) reported palpitations at presentation, which improved or resolved after treating their anemia.[20]

In addition, abnormal pupil size may indicate medication or drug effect or withdrawal. Oral examination should note moist or dry mucous membranes.

Although anxiety is a diagnosis of exclusion and is difficult to diagnose with physical examination alone, patients can often present with a hyperdynamic pulse along with diaphoresis, and abnormal speech patterns.

TESTING (EVALUATION)

Following a thorough history and physical examination, an ECG is warranted, as it has been shown to reveal the cause of palpitations in 27% of patients.[6] Even if the patient is asymptomatic in the office, an ECG may identify many arrhythmias, including, Wolff-Parkinson-White (WPW) syndrome, long QT syndrome, atrioventricular (AV) blocks, atrial fibrillation, premature atrial complexes, and premature ventricular complexes. It can also show evidence of structural heart disease such as atrial enlargement, right ventricular hypertrophy, left ventricular hypertrophy, and prior myocardial infarction.

If the history, physical and/or ECG suggests the possibility of structural heart disease or congestive heart failure, then an echocardiogram should be ordered. This includes anyone with palpitations associated with syncope or presyncope, a family history of HOCM, a murmur or signs of hypervolemia on examination (increased jugular venous pressure, crackles, bilateral lower extremity edema), ECG showing q waves, left bundle branch block, left ventricular hypertrophy, atrial enlargement, AV block, short PR interval and delta waves (WPW syndrome), or prolonged QT interval.[11]

There is no strong evidence to direct laboratory testing in patients presenting with palpitations. Although some articles recommend that all patients presenting with palpitations should have a thyroid stimulating hormone, complete blood count, and basic metabolic panel checked,[9,21] a position paper by the European Heart Rhythm Association states that targeted laboratory testing should be done only when history and physical examination suggest a cause such as hyperthyroidism, anemia, drug use, or pheochromocytoma.[22] Abnormal renal function and derangements of potassium and sodium can cause cardiac arrhythmias. Illicit substances can cause palpitations, making urine toxicology important if there is history or clinical suspicion of drug use.[9,21,22] Based on the relative cost of bloodwork compared with other diagnostic modalities (see **Box 4**), this remains a relatively cost-efficient starting point for the workup of palpitations.[23]

Palpitations lacking a clear diagnosis after performing a history, physical examination, and ECG are classified as "unexplained palpitations." According to the 2017 expert consensus statement by the International Society for Holter and Noninvasive Electrocardiology and the Heart Rhythm Society (ISHNE-HRS), ambulatory ECG monitoring is indicated for patients with unexplained palpitations who meet any of the following criteria displayed in **Box 3** (Class I Recommendation with level of evidence B-R). The American College of Cardiology/American Heart Association guidelines from 1999 recommend ambulatory ECG monitoring to evaluate patients with unexplained recurrent palpitations.[24] There are multiple types of ambulatory ECG monitors including 24- to 48-hour Holter monitors and continuous loop event monitors. The ISHNE-HRS consensus statement gives a Class I recommendation with level of evidence B-NR for doing a 24- to 48-hour Holter monitor when frequent symptomatic events reliably occur within the recording window (daily or more often).[25] In

---

Box 3
Indications for ambulatory electrocardiogram monitoring based on the 2017 consensus statement from the International Society for Holter and Non-invasive Electrocardiology-Heart Rhythm Society in patients with unexplained palpitations

1. When history, physical examination, and 12-lead ECG suggest a possibility of arrhythmia

2. In the setting of diagnosed structural heart disease, family history of sudden cardiac death, or inherited channelopathy with known risk of arrhythmia

3. When patients need reassurance and specific explanation of their symptoms

4. When symptoms warrant therapy and specifics of treatment depend on a formal arrhythmic diagnosis (eg, ablation, antiarrhythmic therapy)

Data from Steinberg JS, Varma N, Cygankiewicz I, et. al. 2017 ISHNE-HRS expert consensus statement on ambulatory ECG and external cardiac monitoring/telemetry.Heart Rhythm. 2017 Jul;14(7):e55-e96.

---

addition, the consensus statement gives a Class I recommendation with level of evidence B-R for doing 15- to 30-day ambulatory ECG monitoring for patients with undefined symptom frequency or symptoms that do not reliably occur every day.

Holter monitors, when worn, record heart rhythms continuously for 24 to 48 hours and are recommended to evaluate unexplained palpitations that occur at least daily. Patients keep a diary of their symptoms during the recording period in order to correlate the time of the symptoms with a particular portion of ECG recording. One study showed 53% of the patients did not experience their presenting symptoms during the 24-hour Holter monitor period, 13% of patients had an arrhythmia correlating with their symptoms, and 34% of patients had their typical presenting symptoms associated with a recording of normal sinus rhythm.[18] The diagnostic yield of a 24-hour Holter monitor for evaluation of palpitations ranges between 5% and 39%.[6,8,26–28] Forty-eight hour Holter monitor did not have a significantly higher diagnostic yield than 24-hour Holter monitoring for detection of maximal ventricular ectopy in patients with coronary artery disease,[29] and it is rarely valuable.

Holter monitors can inadvertently show asymptomatic arrhythmias. One retrospective study reviewing 518 consecutive Holter monitor recordings found that, of those who did not experience their presenting symptoms during the Holter recording period, 56% were found to have an asymptomatic arrhythmia. Furthermore, of the patients who did experience their typical presenting symptoms but had no correlating arrhythmia, 33% were found to have an arrhythmia during their asymptomatic time periods.[18]

Transtelephonic event monitors such as a continuous loop event monitor are worn continuously for 7 to 30 days and will continuously record the heart rhythm. Durable recordings will only be saved and sent to a central station for the few minutes before and after the patient manually activates it. Many of these devices now have an auto-trigger mode that will automatically save data when the heart rate goes greater or less than a certain threshold. Continuous loop event monitors can miss asymptomatic arrhythmias or arrhythmias associated with syncope, as the patient may not activate the recorder during those events. There is another type of transtelephonic event monitor that is not worn continuously but is carried with the patient and placed on the chest when palpitations occur. This often misses the rhythm at the onset of the palpitations.

The diagnostic yield of transtelephonic event monitors for palpitations is 66% to 83%,[8] which is considerably higher than the diagnostic yield of Holter monitors. A study of 147 patients being worked up for cardiac arrhythmia directly compared the diagnostic yield of 24-hour Holter monitor with 2-week continuous event monitor by having the patients wear both simultaneously and then remove the Holter after 24 hours but continue the event monitor for 2 weeks. During the first 24 hours of simultaneous use of both devices 60 arrhythmic events were noted in both devices and 1 arrhythmic event was detected in the Holter but not the event monitor. However, after the first 24 hours once Holter was removed, the continuous event monitor continued and subsequently detected an additional 36 arrhythmic events. There was a total of 61 events identified by Holter and 96 total events identified by 2 week monitor $(P < .001)$.[30]

Zimetbaum and colleagues conducted a prospective cohort study of 105 patients with palpitations referred for continuous event monitor to assess the diagnostic yield and cost of continuous event monitors for each week over a 4-week time period. **Table 3** shows the cost, cost per new diagnosis made, and number of new diagnoses made per patient in each week by continuous loop event monitors in the United States in 1997. The probability of finding a diagnosis over the 4-week time period took the shape of a logarithmic curve that plateaued around week 2 with marginal additional diagnostic yield in weeks 3 and 4.[8] One hundred percent of the "serious diagnoses" made during this study (supraventricular tachycardia, atrial fibrillation/atrial flutter, nonsustained ventricular tachycardia, high-degree heart block) were made within the first 2 weeks of wearing continuous loop event monitors.[8] Thus 2 weeks is considered the optimal duration of continuous loop event monitors for a highest value balance between diagnostic yield and cost. If the 2-week continuous event monitor does not reveal the cause of palpitations in either a high-risk patient or a patient with significant impact on quality of life, then a referral to cardiology is warranted.

A study evaluating syncope workup in Ontario, Canada in 2005 reported the cost (including material, tech/labor, service, overhead, and professional) from Ontario-based fee codes converted to US dollars of various diagnostic testing strategies that are frequently used in the workup of palpitations. The *relative* costs may be applicable to workup of palpitations in the United States and are displayed in **Box 4** rounded to the nearest dollar amount.[23]

The cost per diagnosis is important because once a definitive diagnosis is established, that halts further testing (associated with further diagnostic expenditures) and shifts the focus to appropriate management. Overall, the Holter monitor is

Table 3
Cost, cost per new diagnosis made, and number of new diagnoses made per patient by continuous loop event monitors in the United States in 1997

Length of Time Event Monitor Worn	Cost of Event Monitor in 1997 US Dollars	Cost per New Diagnosis Made in the Additional Time	Number of New Diagnoses Made per Patient during Each Additional Week
Week 1	$102	$98	1.04
Week 2	$96 (+$102 = $198)	$576	0.17
Week 3	$81 (+$198 = $279)	$5832	0.01
Week 4	$81 (+$279 = $360)	No new diagnoses made	0.00

Data from Steinberg JS, Varma N, Cygankiewicz I, et. al. 2017 ISHNE-HRS expert consensus statement on ambulatory ECG and external cardiac monitoring/telemetry.Heart Rhythm. 2017 Jul;14(7):e55-e96.

> **Box 4**
> **Cost of various testing in Ontario, Canada in 2005 in US dollars**
>
> Primary care doctor initial assessment: $49
>
> Primary care doctor follow-up: $25
>
> Emergency room visit: $64
>
> ECG: $21
>
> Bloodwork: $10
>
> 24-h Holter: $103
>
> 48-h Holter: $178
>
> External loop (1 mo): $534
>
> Echocardiogram: $228
>
> Cardiology consult: $103
>
> Electrophysiologic study: $937
>
> Standard treadmill stress test: $142
>
> Stress: MIBI $616
>
> Cardiac catheterization: $462
>
> *Adapted from* Rockx MA, Hoch JS, Klein GJ, et al. Is ambulatory monitoring for "communityac-quired" syncope economically attractive? A cost-effectiveness analysis of a randomized trial of external loop recorders versus Holter monitoring. American Heart Journal. 2005;150(5):1065; with permission.

cheaper but of much lower diagnostic yield, making the event monitor more cost-effective and the ambulatory ECG the test of choice unless palpitations are consistently experienced at least every 24 hours.

Many patients currently use smartwatches or other "wearables," which are consumer grade devices that record heart rate (usually not heart rhythm) by photoplethysmography. Although some of these devices have achieved or are seeking Food and Drug Administration (FDA) "clearance" (considered safe), none of these devices currently have FDA "approval" (endorses evidence of accuracy for medical use). According to the 2017 ISHNE-HRS expert consensus statement on ambulatory ECG and external cardiac monitoring/telemetry, consumer grade devices currently have no medical oversight and should not replace any medically indicated workup at this time.[25] One 2019 study of patients undergoing cardiac rehabilitation showed insufficient concordance of heart rate measurement between various wearable devices and the gold standard of ambulatory ECG monitors.[31] Other studies show some (but not all) models of wearables with high concordance with ambulatory ECGs for heart rate during certain controlled activities (eg, sitting, walking, running, etc.) and overall. However, there is no standard for what level of concordance is considered acceptable for medical use. Of the devices with a high overall concordance with ambulatory ECGs, there was still significant variability in concordance during different types of activities including low concordance during some activities of daily living (chores, brushing teeth) or certain types of exercise (eg, elliptical, cycling). Different devices had different activities during which their measurements were less accurate.[32–36] This is a rapidly evolving field of study with vast potential, given the rapid improvement in device performance during a broad range of activities over the last few years. There are several ongoing studies evaluating the ability of wearables to detect heart rhythm (not just heart rate) abnormalities such as atrial fibrillation and supraventricular arrhythmias.[37,38]

Although these devices have high potential for helping diagnose medically relevant arrhythmias, they may also lead to increased testing and overdiagnosis of asymptomatic benign arrhythmias. Given that Holter monitors have shown a high prevalence of asymptomatic arrhythmias,[18] it is likely that consumer grade wearables will as well. As the technology of commercially available products is exploding, patients may begin to present to their doctors with data from consumer grade devices rather than symptoms. For the time being, clinicians should remain focused on symptom driven evaluation with evidence-based workup dictated by history, physical examination, and ECG, but in the future, wearables may represent an easily accessible and cost-effective way to evaluate palpitations.

Many patients with palpitations can be diagnosed and managed in the outpatient setting without a cardiology referral. If the palpitations are caused by premature atrial or ventricular contractions in the absence of structural heart disease, patients should be reassured about this benign condition, and symptoms can be managed with a beta-blocker, if needed. A longitudinal study demonstrated no increased mortality in patients with frequent premature ventricular contractions without structural heart disease compared with the healthy general population.[29] Red flags that warrant further evaluation (sometimes urgently in the emergency room) include palpitations associated with syncope or presyncope, known or suspected family history of hypertrophic obstructive cardiomyopathy, suspicion of active cardiac ischemia and/or abnormal stress test, and abnormal echocardiogram showing structural heart disease. Practitioners should consider cardiology referral for management of certain arrhythmias diagnosed by primary care provider workup including supraventricular tachycardias, ventricular arrhythmias, or second- or third-degree AV heart blocks. Cardiology referral is also recommended for patients with a negative workup by primary care who are poorly tolerating their symptoms.

SUMMARY

Palpitations are a common chief complaint of patients in the primary care setting, urgent care, emergency department, and cardiology offices. A thorough history is central in helping to narrow down the cause of the palpitations. All components of the patient's history should be addressed, including their personal social and medical history along with their family history. A comprehensive history will help determine who will need further testing and monitoring. Although the physical examination may provide limited additional information, it should be used to guide further workup. There are many options available for additional investigation of the cause of palpitations. Of the available tests, a 2-week continuous loop event monitor has been shown to have the highest diagnostic yield to cost ratio when pursuing ambulatory ECG monitoring.[8] If a patient's symptoms are reportedly occurring at least every 24 hours, a Holter monitor can be used. Currently, there are multiple consumer grade wearable heart monitor devices available to our patients such as smartwatches. Their use and efficacy are still being investigated. At this point their accuracy seems to be variable, and they are likely to provide a lot of clinically irrelevant data. Nevertheless, they do have an exciting potential for medical use in the future and may have the ability to reduce the overall cost of a palpitations workup.

DISCLOSURE

The authors have no conflicts of interest to disclose.

REFERENCES

1. Derogatis LR, Lipman RS, Rickels K, et al. The Hopkins Symptom Checklist (HSCL): a self-report symptom inventory. Behav Sci 1974;19:1–15.
2. Swartz M, Hughes D, George L, et al. Developing a screening index for community studies of somatization disorder. J Psychiatry Res 1986;20:335–43.
3. Kroenke K, Arrington ME, Mangelsdroff AD. The prevalence of symptoms in medical outpatients and the adequacy of therapy. Arch Intern Med 1990;150:1685–9.
4. Mayou R. Chest pain, palpitations and panic. J Psychosom Res 1998;44:53–70.
5. Knudson MP. The natural history of palpitations in a family practice. J Fam Pract 1987;24:357–60.
6. Weber BE, Kapoor WN. Evaluation and outcomes of patients with palpitations. The Am J Med 1996;14(6):138–48.
7. Summerton N, Mann S, Rigby A, et al. New-onset palpitations in general practice: assessing the discriminant value of items within the clinical history. Fam Pract 2001;383–92.
8. Zimetbaum P, Josephson ME. Evaluation of patients with palpitations. New Engl J Med 1998;338(19):1369–73.
9. Wexler R, Pleister A, Raman S. Palpitations: evaluation in the primary care setting. Am Fam Physician 2017;784–9.
10. Borjesson M, Pelliccia A. Incidence and aetiology of sudden cardiac death in young athletes: an international perspective. Br J Sports Med 2009;43(9):644–8.
11. Abbott AV. Diagnostic approach to palpitations. Am Fam Med 2005;71(4):743–50.
12. Walker HK, Hall WD, Hurst JW. Clinical methods: the history, physical, and laboratory examinations. Boston: Butterworths; 1990.
13. Barsky AJ. Somatized psychiatric disorder presenting as palpitations. Arch Intern Med 1996;156(10):1102–8.
14. Chung MK. Vitamins, supplements, herbal medicines, and arrhythmias. Cardiol Rev 2004;12(2):73–84.
15. Deligiannis AP, Kouidi E. Cardiovascular adverse effects of doping in sports. Hellenic J Cardiol 2012;53(6):447–57.
16. Patel J, Rifai MA, Scheuner MT, et al. Basic vs more complex definitions of family history in the prediction of coronary heart disease: the multi-ethnic study of atherosclerosis. Mayo Clinic Proc 2018;93(9):1213–23.
17. Raj SR. The Postural Tachycardia Syndrome (POTS): pathophysiology, diagnosis & management. Indian Pacing Electrophysiol J 2006;6(2):84–99.
18. Zeldis SM, Levine BJ, Michelson EL, et al. Cardiovascular complaints. Correlation with cardiac arrhythmias on 24-hour electrocardiographic monitoring. Chest 1980;78:456–61.
19. Noah MS, Sulimani RA. Prolapse of the mitral valve in hyperthyroid patients in Saudi Arabia. Int J Cardiol 1988;19(2):217-223.
20. Dhamangaonkar MP, Golwalkar JK. Directory of Open Access Journals. Journal of Evidence Based Medicine and Healthcare. 2017. Available at: https://doaj.org/article/bee966d94197479ebde8c295d5c05097. Accessed February 5, 2020.
21. Gale CP, Camm AJ. Assessment of palpitations. BMJ 2016;352.
22. Raviele A, Giada F, Bergfeldt L, et al. Management of patients with palpitations: a position paper from the European Heart Rhythm Association. Europace 2011;13(7):920–34.
23. Rockx MA, Hoch JS, Klein GJ, et al. Is ambulatory monitoring for "community-acquired" syncope economically attractive? A cost-effectiveness analysis of a

randomized trial of external loop recorders versus Holter monitoring. Am Heart J 2005;150(5):1065.

24. Crawford MH, Bernstein SJ, Deedwania PC, et al. ACC/AHA guidelines for ambulatory electrocardiography: executive summary and recommendations. A report of the American College of Cardiology/American Heart Association task force on practice guidelines (committee to revise the guidelines for ambulatory electrocardiography). Circulation 1999;100:886–9.

25. Steinberg JS, Varma N, Cygankiewicz I, et al. 2017 ISHNE-HRS expert consensus statement on ambulatory ECG and external cardiac monitoring/telemetry. Heart Rhythm 2017;14(7):55–96.

26. Olson JA, Fouts AM, Padanilam BJ, et al. Utility of mobile cardiac outpatient telemetry for the diagnosis of palpitations, presyncope, syncope, and the assessment of therapy efficacy. J Cardiovasc Electrophysiol 2007;18:473–7.

27. Ritter MA, Kochhäuser S, Duning T, et al. Occult atrial fibrillation in cryptogenic stroke: detection by 7-day electrocardiogram versus implantable cardiac monitors. Stroke 2013;44:1449–52.

28. Rothman SA, Laughlin JC, Seltzer J, et al. The diagnosis of cardiac arrhythmias: a prospective multi-center randomized study comparing mobile cardiac outpatient telemetry versus standard loop event monitoring. J Cardiovasc Electrophysiol 2007;18:241–7.

29. Kennedy HL, Chandra V, Sayther KL, et al. Effectiveness of increasing hours of continuous ambulatory electrocardiography in detecting maximal ventricular ectopy: continuous 48 hour study of patients with coronary heart disease and normal subjects. Am J Cardiol 1978;42:925–30.

30. Barrett PM, Komatireddy R, Haaser S, et al. Comparison of 24-hour Holter monitoring with 14-day novel adhesive patch electrocardiographic monitoring. Am J Med 2017;127:95.e11–7.

31. Etiwy M, Akhrass Z, Gillinov L, et al. Accuracy of wearable heart rate monitors in cardiac rehabilitation. Cardiovasc Diagn Ther 2019;9(3):262–71.

32. Nelson BW, Allen NB. Accuracy of consumer wearable heart rate measurement during an ecologically valid 24-hour period: intraindividual validation study. JMIR Mhealth Uhealth 2019;7(3):e10828.

33. Wang R, Blackburn G, Desai M, et al. Accuracy of wrist-worn heart rate monitors. JAMA Cardiol 2017;2:104–6.

34. Gillinov S, Etiwy M, Wang R, et al. Variable accuracy of wearable heart rate monitors during aerobic exercise. Med Sci Sports Exerc 2017;49:1697–703.

35. Parak J, Korhonen I. Evaluation of wearable consumer heart rate monitors based on photopletysmography. Annu Int Conf IEEE Eng Med Biol Soc. Chicago, IL: August 26-30, 2014;2014:3670-3. doi:10.1109/EMBC.2014.6944419. PMID: 25570787.

36. Shcherbina A, Mattsson C, Waggott D, et al. Accuracy in wrist-worn, sensor-based measurements of heart rate and energy expenditure in a diverse cohort. J Pers Med 2017;7:3.

37. Cheung C, Krahn A, Andrade J. The emerging role of wearable technologies in detection of arrhythmia. Can J Cardiol 2018;34(8):1083–7.

38. Bumgarner JM, Lambert CT, Hussein AA, et al. Automated atrial fibrillation detection algorithm using smartwatch technology. J Am Coll Cardiol 2018;71:2381–8.

Solving the Problem of Insomnia in Clinical Practice

Adrienne F. Willard, MD[a],*, Allison H. Ferris, MD[b]

KEYWORDS

- Insomnia • Poor sleep • Sleep disorder • Primary care • Outpatient medicine

KEY POINTS

- Chronic insomnia affects 50 to 70 million Americans annually and is a common reason patients seek outpatient primary care.
- There is good evidence to support the use of cognitive behavioral therapy for insomnia (CBT-I) to treat chronic insomnia as first-line therapy. The use of pharmacotherapy as the first line to treat chronic insomnia should be avoided.
- When pharmacotherapy is necessary to augment CBT-I, use for the shortest duration possible, ideally less than 5 weeks.
- If pharmacotherapy is still needed after this duration, shared decision making regarding the risks and benefits of ongoing medication use is imperative.
- Selection of appropriate medication is highly individualized.

INTRODUCTION

Insomnia is a common condition that affects everyone at some point in their lives, whether it be short-term insomnia or chronic insomnia. Up to 50% of people report intermittent sleep disturbances, whereas chronic sleep disturbances affect between 50 and 70 million Americans.[1–3] Data from the Centers for Disease Control and Prevention reveal that insomnia affected 19.2% (46.2 million) adults in 2012, an increase from 17.5% (37.5 million) in 2002.[4] The human body needs sleep in order for proper functioning, so insomnia can have negative effects on health as well as productivity. The National Safety Council estimates the cost to employers to be $1200 to $3100 per year,[5] resulting in big-picture estimates of between $30 and $136 billion per year in direct and indirect costs, including visits to health care providers, medications, increased accidents, and lost work productivity.[3,5] Insomnia accounts for 5.5 million outpatient visits annually[6]: primary care providers must be knowledgeable in diagnosing and managing this common condition.

[a] Drexel University College of Medicine, 2900 West Queen Lane, Philadelphia, PA 19129, USA;
[b] Charles E. Schmidt College of Medicine, 800 Meadows Rd, Boca Raton, FL 33486, USA
* Corresponding author.
E-mail address: afw38@drexel.edu

Med Clin N Am 105 (2021) 107–116
https://doi.org/10.1016/j.mcna.2020.09.006
0025-7125/21/© 2020 Elsevier Inc. All rights reserved.

medical.theclinics.com

DEFINITION

According to the *International Classification of Sleep Disorders, Third Edition* (from the American Academy of Sleep Medicine [AASM]), insomnia is divided into 3 categories: chronic insomnia disorder, short-term insomnia disorder, and other insomnia disorder.[7] Similarly, the *Diagnostic and Statistical Manual of Mental Disorders* (Fifth Edition) reclassified primary insomnia as insomnia disorder and emphasizes that insomnia can occur in isolation or in combination with other comorbidities. When insomnia is a comorbidity, it is not treated as separate from coexisting mental illnesses or medical conditions; therefore, the treatment of insomnia addresses not only the sleep component but also the underlying conditions.[8] Short-term insomnia disorder is defined as lasting less than 3 months (usually days to weeks) and has identifiable triggers or stressors, including physical, psychological, psychosocial, or interpersonal.[9] Chronic insomnia by definition lasts greater than 3 months, happens at least 3 nights per week, and is associated with compromised daytime functioning.[6,8,9] There are a variety of signs or symptoms that constitute compromised daytime functioning, including fatigue, poor concentration, inability to function in school/work/social situations, mood disturbances or variability, daytime sleepiness, decreased motivation or energy, increased errors or accidents, behavioral issues, and ongoing worry/preoccupation with sleep.[7,9] If a patient has features of insomnia but does not meet the criteria for either short-term or chronic insomnia, they fall into the other insomnia category.

PATHOPHYSIOLOGY

Adults need between 7 and 9 hours of sleep per night for optimal health.[1] Sleep consists of 2 states: REM (rapid eye movement) and NREM (nonrapid eye movement). The body cycles between these states throughout the night, culminating in 4 to 5 REM periods, which account for about one-fourth of the total night's sleep.[1,10] The deepest sleep occurs during NREM in the first few hours of the night.[1,10] The sleep-wake cycle is regulated by circuits in the brain that make up the arousal system and the sleep-promoting system; these systems use monoaminergic, glutamatergic, and cholinergic neurons to activate various parts of the brain or GABAergic neurons to inhibit the arousal areas.[1]

Several things can disrupt the sleep cycle, including normal age-related changes, medications, alcohol, and psychiatric disorders. For example, depression can cause an earlier onset of REM sleep as well as a shift of REM activity to the first half of the night, thereby interfering with the timing and amount of deep NREM sleep.[10] Older adults naturally see a decrease in the deep NREM sleep and an increase in wakeful time during the night, leading to an overall decrease in sleep time.[1,10] Alcohol leads to disruption of the sleep cycle by blocking REM sleep as well as disrupting the natural circadian rhythm and causing an increase in vivid dreams and awakenings.[10] Various medications can interfere with the neurotransmitters in the arousal or sleep-promoting systems of the brain and subsequently cause insomnia.[1]

DIAGNOSIS

A directed history is the key to successfully diagnosing insomnia. Insomnia is dissatisfaction with sleep quality or quantity; by definition, it is subjective in nature and requires careful questioning to best understand the issue and to ultimately tailor the best treatment plan.[11,12] A sleep history must catalog sleep habits and outcomes as well as look for risk factors for insomnia.[1,2,12] Sleep habits are highly individualized, and a provider must inquire about a patient's behaviors surrounding bed and sleep, events during sleep, and their relationship with sleep.[12] Some suggested questions are found in **Box 1**. When asking about sleep habits, it is important to ask usual bedtime and wake time in addition to asking how long it takes for the person to fall asleep. Sleep latency is the amount of time it takes to get from full wakefulness to sleep. In non-sleep-deprived individuals, this value is typically 15 to 20 minutes, whereas shorter latency times indicate sleep deprivation. A detailed sleep diary for 24 hours and/or 1 to 2 weeks can provide robust information regarding sleep habits, satisfaction, and effect on daytime function.[1,9,12]

A useful and validated tool for practitioners to obtain a standard history is the Pittsburgh Sleep Quality Index (PSQI) questionnaire. This questionnaire includes a series of questions about sleep quality, latency, duration, efficiency, sleep disturbances, use of medications, and daytime dysfunction. The PSQI scoring ranges from 0 to 21 points with anything greater than 5 indicative of a sleep disturbance.[9]

Several important areas must also be investigated with thorough questioning, including comorbid psychological or psychiatric disorders, medication (both prescription and nonprescription) history, and other medical conditions.[1,10] Eighty percent of individuals with psychiatric disorders, including anxiety, depression, and mania, complains of insomnia as a symptom.[1] Medications, including antidepressants (specifically the selective serotonin reuptake inhibitors and serotonin-norepinephrine reuptake inhibitors), stimulants, corticosteroids, albuterol, caffeine, alcohol, and nicotine, can all negatively impact sleep and sleep satisfaction.[1] Clinicians should attempt to address underlying medical conditions that may be contributing to sleep disturbances and viewed as a risk factor for insomnia. These medical conditions might include persistent pain, cardiac or respiratory failure, and chronic inflammatory conditions, such as arthritis or inflammatory bowel disorder.[12]

A diagnostic workup for insomnia is not necessary unless there is concern for another sleep disorder, such as restless leg syndrome (RLS), periodic limb movement disorder, narcolepsy, or obstructive sleep apnea (OSA).[1,9,11] There are some high-yield, high-specificity historical details that can help identify these alternative diagnoses. For example, if a patient complains of creeping discomfort in calves or feet that triggers an irresistible urge to move the limbs, in particular, at night or while at rest, RLS should be considered.[1] Similarly, a history consistent with cataplexy, emotionally triggered transient muscle weakness lasting usually less than 2 minutes, should prompt the consideration of narcolepsy.[13] Finally, a history of nocturnal gasping or

---

Box 1
Suggested questions for obtaining a sleep history

1. Tell me about your bedtime routine, including what time you typically go to bed and what time you wake up. Do you deviate from this on the weekends?

2. Do you usually take naps in the daytime?

3. Do you tend to use your bed for any of the following: reading, studying, watching TV, playing on your phone/tablet, working, and so forth?

4. Do you (or your bed partner) ever notice any of the following: snoring, leg movements, restlessness/tossing and turning, nightmares, frequent waking, and so forth?

5. Do you have any specific emotions about sleep (ie, do you sleep when you're mad or sad, do you sleep when you're anxious, do you feel upset when you go to sleep, do you have any fears about sleep, and so forth)?

choking and recurrent morning headaches should trigger clinicians to investigate a diagnosis of OSA.

If sleep complaints suggest chronic insomnia after a careful history, there are several criteria that should be met. These criteria defined by the AASM are listed in **Table 1.**

TREATMENT

Treatment of acute insomnia should directly address the triggers or stressors once identified since the insomnia typically resolves when the cause is eliminated or mitigated. Treatment includes efforts to ameliorate or limit the triggers, providing reassurance that symptoms of insomnia are an appropriate reaction to circumstances and should resolve, and educating patients on proper sleep hygiene.[12] If necessary, a short-term course of sedatives, such as benzodiazepine receptor agonists or benzodiazepines (BZDs), may be appropriate.[14] Reassessment every few weeks is important to ensure the patient is not developing chronic insomnia or maladaptive responses to the insomnia, including dependence on medications.

In general, there are 2 arms of therapy to treat chronic insomnia: psychological and pharmacologic. The first-line therapy for treatment of chronic insomnia is psychological therapy, primarily as cognitive behavioral therapy targeted for insomnia (CBT-I).[2,11,12,16–18] CBT-I is multifaceted and incorporates behavioral interventions (such as sleep restriction, stimulus control, and relaxation techniques) and educational interventions (such as teaching about sleep hygiene) with cognitive restructuring (reframing the patient's ideas or preconceived notions about sleep).[2,11,12,16–19] Practically, this content can be delivered over 2 to 8 sessions weekly by a qualified health care professional in person via either individual or group setting or virtually through the Internet.[6,12] The AASM has published guidelines that support the effectiveness of psychological and behavioral interventions, stimulus control therapy, relaxation training, and sleep restriction to treat chronic insomnia with a high degree of clinical certainty.[16]

Multiple studies have demonstrated that CBT-I is effective. A metaanalysis published in 2015 demonstrated the CBT-I reduced both time to sleep onset (by 19 minutes) and the amount of wakefulness after sleep onset (by 26 minutes) and that the

---

Table 1
Diagnostic criteria for chronic insomnia disorder

The diagnostic criteria for chronic insomnia disorder from the International Classification of Sleep Disorder the 3rd edition states the 6 criteria must be met. The first criteria is the patient or their caregiver reporting one or more of the following: difficulty initiating sleep, difficulty maintaining sleep, waking up earlier than desired, resistance to going to bed on an appropriate schedule, or difficulty sleeping without parent or guarding intervention. The second criteria requires demonstration of daytime dysfunction as one or more of the following: a history of fatigue or malaise; attention, concentration or memory impairment; impaired alert , family, occupations or academic performance; mood disturbance; daytime sleepiness; behavioral problems; reduced motivation or initiative, proneness to errors or accidents, or concerns about dissatisfaction with sleep. The third criteria is a reported sleep-wake complaints cannot be explained by inadequate opportunity or circumstances for sleep. The fourth criteria is the finding that the sleep disturbances and associated daytime symptoms occur at least 3 times per week. The fifth criteria is the presence of sleep disturbance for at least 3 months. The final criteria that must be met is the fact that the sleep-wake disturbances cannot be better explained by another sleep disorder.[15]

effects were sustained up to 12 months after treatment.[12] In another study, CBT-I was found to have sustained effectiveness at 6 months with no major side effects.[6]

This behavioral approach to initial therapy is endorsed by multiple professional societies, including the American College of Physicians (ACP), AASM, and the American Academy of Family Physicians.[6,18,20] It is critical, however, to acknowledge the limitations of this treatment approach, specifically in areas such as access to care (limited professionals to deliver treatment), cost (to patient), and potential for drop out due to long duration.[14,21] There is a variant of CBT-I called brief behavioral therapy for insomnia, which combines stimulus control with sleep restriction over a shorter duration of treatment that has also seen some success in improving sleep outcomes.[16,21] This therapy may provide a real-world solution for clinicians and patients who cannot or will not complete a more complete CBT-I treatment approach.

Although nondrug therapy should be the emphasis of treatment, a multimodal approach is often needed because of lack of or partial response to psychological treatments.[8] The ACP recommends a shared decision-making approach when adding pharmacologic therapy when CBT-I alone is unsuccessful.[12,18]

There are several classes of medications in the armamentarium to consider for patients with insomnia. These medications include hypnotics, sedating antidepressants, orexin antagonists, melatonin agonists, antihistamines, and antipsychotics. All medications have side effects and abuse potential that must be considered in each patient before initiating therapy. A summary of the Food and Drug Administration (FDA)-approved agents is located in **Table 2**.[8,14,18,20,22,23]

Hypnotics

The "Z-drugs" are often the first class of medications that clinicians select for chronic insomnia. These medications are BZD receptor agonists and include zolpidem, zaleplon, and eszopiclone; they reduce sleep latency by about 20 minutes.[8,20] Eszopiclone and zolpidem both improve sleep maintenance as well.[20] Zolpidem comes in immediate release, extended release, and sublingual formulations.[22] The immediate release option allows for good results with reducing sleep latency and increasing total sleep time, whereas the extended release formulation only increases the risk of next day sedation but does not appear to offer additional benefits.[8] The sublingual formulation is specifically designed for middle-of-the-night awakenings.[20] Zaleplon has a slightly shorter half-life and is also useful for patients with nighttime awakenings.[8] Eszopiclone has a unique side effect of potentially causing a distortion in the sense of taste, so this should be mentioned to patients if it is prescribed.[8] All hypnotics carry the risk of next day sedation, especially more prominent in those drugs with longer half-lives, such as eszopiclone. In general, hypnotics should only be a short-term measure.[12]

BZDs act on GABA receptors, and GABA inhibits the arousal system of the brain.[1] Although many different BZDs are prescribed by clinicians for insomnia, only five are approved by the FDA for treatment of insomnia (estazolam, flurazepam, quazepam, triazolam, and temazepam),[24] and only triazolam and temazepam are recommended by the AASM for use in chronic insomnia.[20] Triazolam at a dose of 0.25 mg is recommended for improving sleep onset, whereas temazepam at a dose of 15 mg is recommended for both improving sleep onset and sleep maintenance.[20] The ACP in developing their clinical practice guidelines, however, found insufficient evidence to support use of BZDs for treatment of insomnia.[18]

Sedating Antidepressants

Because of the high prevalence of insomnia in depressed patients, the use of sedating antidepressants may serve a dual purpose. Trazodone is a heterocyclic

Table 2
Common medications for insomnia treatment

Medication	Usual Dosage	Utility	Clinical Consideration[a]	Cost[b]
BZD-receptor agonists				
Zolpidem	5 mg, 10 mg 6.25, 12.5 mg (CR)	Sleep onset and maintenance	Parasomnias (eg, sleep eating, sleepwalking, nightmares, confusional arousals)	$16
Zolpidem sublingual	1.75, 3.5 mg	Nocturnal awakenings	Parasomnias	$80
Eszopiclone	1, 2, 3 mg	Sleep onset and maintenance	Parasomnias, dysgeusia, next day sedation[a]	$14
Zaleplon	5, 10 mg	Sleep onset and nocturnal awakenings	Parasomnias	$12
Benzodiazepines				
Triazolam	0.125, 0.25 mg	Sleep onset	Addictive potential, anterograde amnesia, respiratory depression	$36
Temazepam	7.5, 15, 22.5, 30 mg	Sleep onset and maintenance	Addictive potential, anterograde amnesia, respiratory depression	$36
Antidepressants				
Doxepin	3, 6 mg	Sleep maintenance	Parasomnias, suicidal ideation, SIADH, serotonin syndrome	$109
Orexin-antagonists				
Suvorexant	5, 10, 15, 20 mg	Sleep onset and maintenance	Moderate addictive potential, next day impairment, parasomnias	$369
Melatonin agonists				
Ramelteon	8 mg	Sleep onset	No major concerns	$90
Antihistamines				
Diphenhydramine	25, 50 mg	Not recommended by AASM	Urinary retention, avoid in glaucoma, tachyphylaxis with chronic use	$2
Doxylamine	25 mg	Not recommended by AASM	Urinary retention, avoid in glaucoma, tachyphylaxis with chronic use	$5

Abbreviations: CR, controlled release; SIADH, syndrome of inappropriate antidiuretic hormone secretion.

[a] All hypnotics have a risk of next day sedation associated with them. Some with longer half-lives have greater relative risk of this.

[b] Estimated retail price of 1 month's treatment at the lowest dose based on information obtained at http://www.goodrx.com for prescription medications (accessed April 29, 2020).

Data from Refs.[8,14,18,20,22,23]

antidepressant that is sedating. It has a low abuse potential and is cost-efficient, which also makes it appealing[1]; however, it is not recommended by the AASM given the lack of evidence of efficacy and the potential for harm outweighing benefits.[20] Doxepin is a tricyclic antidepressant that has a strong H1-agonist effect that leads to its sedating properties that help with insomnia. When doxepin is used for depression, the dose is typically 25 to 300 mg daily; however, the dose for insomnia is much lower, only 3 to 6 mg daily,[20] and these doses are only available as brand-name medications, which drives up cost.

Orexin Antagonists

Orexin is a neurotransmitter found in the hypothalamus that reinforces awakeness.[1] One of the newest agents approved for the treatment of insomnia is suvorexant, an orexin-antagonist that blocks the effects of the arousal neurotransmitter. Suvorexant at the suggested doses of 10, 15, or 20 mg is recommended for the treatment of sleep maintenance insomnia.[20] It has a very minimal side-effect profile, which makes it an appealing option for many patients.

Melatonin Agonists

Melatonin is a hormone that has some effects on sleep habits. It is secreted by the pineal gland, and its secretion is inhibited by ambient light; therefore, melatonin supplementation may help in individuals who attempt to sleep during the daytime (such as shift-workers) or in patients who have central nervous system issues, such as spinal cord injuries or Parkinson disease.[1] Ramelteon, a melatonin agonist, at a dose of 8 mg is recommended as an agent to help improve sleep onset.[20] The side-effect profile is minimal and was found to be no different than placebo; hence, it is thought to be a very safe agent for use, even in elderly patients.[20] Unfortunately, there is no evidence to support the use of over-the-counter melatonin products (usual dose 2–5 mg).[6,20]

Other Agents

Antihistamines are the active ingredient in most over-the- counter sleep aids, such as diphenhydramine and doxylamine. They are approved by the FDA given their relatively acceptable safety profile[24]; however, there is no evidence to support their efficacy, and therefore, they are not recommended by the AASM for use in chronic insomnia.[6,20]

Several other classes of medications are sometimes prescribed to patients with insomnia because of their side-effect profile (specifically the sedating effect of the drug). Examples of these include gabapentin, pregabalin, risperidone, olanzapine, and quetiapine.[22] The AASM does not recommend the use of these agents, given the paucity of evidence and lack of clinical trials specific to insomnia.[20] In some patients, however, who have underlying conditions for which those medications are indicated (neuropathy, psychiatric illnesses), the sleep-effect benefits may be helpful.

Duration of Treatment

Ideally, medications should be used for a short duration, such as 4 to 5 weeks, and then treatment should focus on using the skills learned during CBT-I.[18] Of all the above medications, only zolpidem, eszopiclone, and suvorexant improved outcomes in short-term studies of 3 months or less, so there is limited evidence for long-term efficacy.[6] Despite the evidence and guidelines, however, there is a subset of individuals who have been on long-term hypnotic medications to treat their chronic insomnia. Providers should be encouraged by the evidence that supports the use of psychological and behavioral interventions to treat this population as well. The AASM found 4 randomized controlled trials of moderate to high clinical evidence to support the addition of behavioral therapy to long-standing pharmacologic treatment.[16] Ultimately, whatever treatment is selected for an individual, clinicians must be certain to address anxiety about sleep, maladaptive behaviors around sleep, and fear of further disruption of sleep.[12]

LONG-TERM CONSEQUENCES/SEQUELAE

Left untreated, chronic insomnia can have a deleterious effect on patients. Untreated insomnia increases the risk of developing anxiety, depression, hypertension, and diabetes.[12] In addition, it has been found that persistent insomnia with depression is associated with suicide.[19]

As previously stated, there are no side effects from CBT-I, but it does not always lead to the desired response and improvement in sleep quality and quantity; thus, the use of pharmacotherapy for longer durations than the suggested 4 to 5 weeks may be warranted. The chronic use of Z-drugs must involve a discussion and shared decision making regarding the potential for increased risk of cardiovascular events, cancers, and all-cause mortality even though results about these risks have been mixed in studies.[8] These drugs also have a boxed warning from the FDA for the risk of sleepwalking, sleep eating, sleep driving, and other activities.[25] Observational studies have shown an increase in dementia and fractures with hypnotic drugs.[6,18] Treating elderly patients with pharmacotherapy brings the added risks of falls into the discussion, as all sedating medications have this potential side effect. BZDs have a risk of developing addiction after even only a few weeks of treatment, and the risk of developing a dependence is high. In addition, 15% to 40% of users report severe withdrawal symptoms after cessation of BZDs.[22] All of these risks and sequelae must be taken into consideration when choosing pharmacologic therapy for chronic insomnia. Ultimately, providers must consider the long-term effects of being sleep deprived and weigh them against the potential harms of treatments when treating chronic insomnia.

SUMMARY

Insomnia is a common condition encountered in primary care clinics that can have deleterious effects on the patient. Clinicians must be adept at identifying the problem, searching for comorbid conditions, and developing a treatment plan. Each patient requires an individualized approach, ideally focusing on identifying and managing triggers or stressors, followed by psychological interventions, only culminating in pharmacologic treatment if needed. Patients should be reevaluated regularly for side effects, harms, and long-term sequelae of both the insomnia and any treatments. Shared decision making is critical for success in managing this common symptom in outpatient practice.

CLINICS CARE POINTS

- Cognitive Behavioral Therapy for Insomnia (CBT-I) is the cornerstone for treatment of insomnia.
- Pharmacotherapy should be used for the shortest duration possible at the lowest effective dose.

DISCLOSURE

Neither Dr A.F. Willard nor Dr A.H. Ferris have any conflicts of interest to disclose.

REFERENCES

1. Scammell TE, Saper CB, Czeisler CA. Sleep disorders. In: Jameson J, Fauci AS, Kasper DL, et al. editors. Harrison's principles of internal medicine, 20e New York: McGraw-Hill. Available at: http://accessmedicine.mhmedical.com.ezproxy.fau.edu/content.aspx?bookid=2129&sectionid=192344545. Accessed April 19, 2020.

2. Schutte-Rodin S, Broch L, Buysse D, et al. Clinical guideline for the evaluation and management of chronic insomnia in adults. J Clin Sleep Med 2008;4(5):487–504.

3. Klemas N. Clinical economics: insomnia. Med Econ 2015;92(6):24–5.

4. Ford ES, Cunningham TJ, Giles WH, et al. Trends in insomnia and excessive daytime sleepiness among US adults from 2002 to 2012. Sleep Med 2015;16(3):372–8.

5. Cost of sleepiness too pricey to ignore. AASM press release. 2018. Available at: https://aasm.org/cost-sleepiness-pricey-ignore/. Accessed April 20, 2020.

6. Salisbury-Afshar E. Management of insomnia disorder in adults. Am Fam Physician 2018;98(5):319–22.

7. Sateia MJ. International classification of sleep disorders-third edition. Highlights and modifications. Chest 2014;146(5):1387–94.

8. Bragg S, Benich JJ, Christian N, et al. Updates in insomnia diagnosis and treatment. Int J Psychiatry Med 2019;54(4–5):275–89.

9. Bonnet MH, Arand DL. Evaluation and diagnosis of insomnia in adults. UpToDate. Available at: https://www.uptodate.com/contents/evaluation-and-diagnosis-of-insomnia-in-adults/print?search=insomnia&source=search_result&selectedTitle=3~150&usage_type=default&display_rank=3. Accessed April 18, 2020.

10. Raj KS, Williams N, DeBattista C. Sleep-wake disorders. In: Papadakis MA, McPhee SJ, Rabow MW, editors. Current medical diagnosis and treatment 2020 New York: McGraw-Hill. Available at: http://accessmedicine.mhmedical.com.ezproxy.fau.edu/content.aspx?bookid=2683&sectionid=225133422. Accessed April 25, 2020.

11. Winkleman JW. Insomnia disorder. N Engl J Med 2015;373:1437–44.

12. Cunnington D, Junge M. Chronic insomnia: diagnosis and non-pharmacological management. BMJ 2016;355:i5819.

13. Scamell TE. Clinical features and diagnosis of narcolepsy in adults. UpToDate. Available at: https://www.uptodate.com/contents/clinical-features-and-diagnosis-of-narcolepsy-in-adults?search=narcolepsy&sectionRank=2&usage_type=default&anchor=H23706075&source=machineLearning&selectedTitle=1~118&display_rank=1#H23706075. Accessed April 29, 2020.

14. Winkleman JW. Overview of the treatment of insomnia in adults. UpToDate. Available at: https://www.uptodate.com/contents/overview-of-the-treatment-of-insomnia-in-adults?search=insomnia&topicRef=7676&source=see_link#H3610382671. Accessed April 27, 2020.

15. American Academy of Sleep Medicine. International Classification of Sleep Disorders. 3rd ed. Darien, IL: American Academy of Sleep Medicine; 2014.

16. Morgenthaler T, Kramer M, Alessi C, et al. Practice parameters for the psychological and behavioral treatment of insomnia: an update. An American Academy of Sleep Medicine report. Sleep 2006;29(11):1415–9.

17. Trauer JM, Qian MY, Doyle JS, et al. Cognitive behavioral therapy for chronic insomnia: a systematic review and meta-analysis. Ann Intern Med 2015;163: 191–204.
18. Qaseem A, Kansagara D, Forciea MA, et al. for the Clinical Guidelines Committee of the American College of Physicians. Management of chronic insomnia disorder in adults: a clinical practice guideline from the American College of Physicians. Ann Intern Med 2016;165(2):125–33.
19. Haynes P. Application of cognitive behavioral therapies for comorbid insomnia and depression. Sleep Med Clin 2015;10:77–84.
20. Sateia MJ, Buysse DJ, Krystal AD, et al. Clinical practice guideline for the pharmacologic treatment of chronic insomnia in adults: an American Academy of Sleep Medicine clinical practice guideline. J Clin Sleep Med 2017;13(2):307–49.
21. Provider fact sheet: brief behavioral treatment for insomnia (BBT-I). Available at: https://j2vjt3dnbra3ps7ll1clb4q2-wpengine.netdna-ssl.com/wp-content/uploads/2019/03/ProviderFS_BBTI_18.pdf. Accessed April 27, 2020.
22. Matheson E, Hainer BL. Insomnia: pharmacologic therapy. Am Fam Physician 2017;96(1):29–35.
23. Hirsch M. Tricyclic and tetracyclic drugs: pharmacology, administration, and side effects. UpToDate. Available at: https://www.uptodate.com/contents/tricyclic-and-tetracyclic-drugs-pharmacology-administration-and-side-effects?search=doxepin&source=search_result&selectedTitle=2~66&usage_type=default&display_rank=1. Accessed April 28, 2020.
24. Sleep disorder (sedative-hypnotic) drug information. Food and Drug Administration. Available at: https://www.fda.gov/drugs/postmarket-drug-safety-information-patients-and-providers/sleep-disorder-sedative-hypnotic-drug-information. Accessed April 28, 2020.
25. FDA adds boxed warning for risk of serious injuries caused by sleepwalking with certain prescription insomnia medications. Drug Safety Communication, Food and Drug Administration. 2019. Available at: https://www.fda.gov/drugs/drug-safety-and-availability/fda-adds-boxed-warning-risk-serious-injuries-caused-sleepwalking-certain-prescription-insomnia. Accessed April 28, 2020.

Outpatient Evaluation of Knee Pain

Natalie Farha, MD[a],*, Abby Spencer, MD, MS[a,b], Megan McGervey, MD[a,c]

KEYWORDS

- Outpatient knee • Knee pain • Knee exam • Osteoarthritis • Ligamentous tear
- Meniscal injury

KEY POINTS

- Knee pain is one of the most common outpatient complaints.
- A careful history and physical examination are crucial to the diagnosis and management of knee pain.
- Careful consideration should be made before ordering imaging for acute knee pain.
- Conservative management of chronic knee pain owing to osteoarthritis includes weight reduction, physical therapy, and pain control.

APPROACH TO OUTPATIENT KNEE PAIN
Introduction

Knee pain is present in up to 20% of the adult general population and can be significantly debilitating to patients. Six percent of patients presenting to an adult primary care clinic with a symptomatic complaint report knee pain, and many of these visits result in diagnostic imaging and specialty referrals.[1] Taking a detailed history, including mechanism of injury, can help clinicians determine whether the knee pain is a musculoskeletal problem or whether it is part of a systemic illness. If the pain stems from a musculoskeletal problem, a thorough physical examination can help localize the source of inflammation or injury to further determine if imaging, physical therapy, operative repair, or specialty referral is necessary. By following a systematic approach to evaluating knee pain, including a thorough history, a detailed understanding of knee anatomy, a complete physical examination, and, appropriate diagnostic imaging, physicians are able to make the correct diagnosis and formulate an appropriate therapeutic strategy for patients.

[a] Internal Medicine, Cleveland Clinic, Main Campus G10, 9500 Euclid Avenue, G10, Cleveland, OH 44107, USA; [b] Internal Medicine Residency Program, CCLCM of Case Western Reserve University, Cleveland Clinic, 9501 Euclid Avenue, Cleveland, OH 44195, USA; [c] Internal Medicine Residency Program, Department of Internal Medicine, Cleveland Clinic, 9500 Euclid Ave, NA-10, Cleveland, OH 44195, USA
* Corresponding author.
E-mail address: farhan@ccf.org

Med Clin N Am 105 (2021) 117–136
https://doi.org/10.1016/j.mcna.2020.08.017
0025-7125/21/Published by Elsevier Inc.

medical.theclinics.com

Knee Anatomy

An anatomic understanding of the knee provides a basis for identifying the various injury patterns that are typically seen by clinicians. The knee obtains most of its stability from the 4 ligaments surrounding the joint: the anterior cruciate ligament (ACL), posterior cruciate ligament (PCL), medial collateral ligament (MCL), and lateral collateral ligament (LCL). The medial and lateral menisci are crescent-shaped fibrocartilages that are attached to the tibial plateau at the edge of the articulating surfaces of the femur and tibia. They increase joint stability and provide lubrication and shock absorption for the knee joint space. The extensor mechanism of the knee is facilitated by coordination of the patella, patellar tendon, quadriceps tendon, and quadriceps muscle[2] (**Fig. 1**).

Categorizing Knee Pain

Is the pain acute or chronic?

The determination of acute versus chronic knee pain is very important. Acute pain is defined as pain lasting less than 6 weeks' duration, whereas chronic pain is pain lasting longer than 6 weeks. Sometimes, patients may describe chronic pain that has acutely worsened (acute on chronic pattern), which suggests overuse injury that may be newly exacerbated by an increase in activity. In addition, pain may present as sudden-onset pain that has been present for greater than 6 weeks; although technically, this is "chronic pain," it has an acute onset, so the physician should further inquire about the onset and mechanism of injury.

Is the pain traumatic or nontraumatic?

Next, the physician must inquire if the pain is from an injury, which is typically easy to ascertain from the history. Trauma does not necessarily have to be from direct contact; some common causes of noncontact trauma are running, jumping, slipping on ice without a fall, plant and pivot, uneven terrain, or squatting. Especially in older

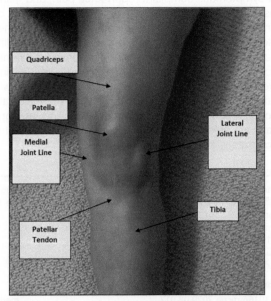

Fig. 1. Knee anatomy.

adults, major injury may result from seemingly minor traumas, so it is important to consider patient demographics and overall functional status when trying to make a diagnosis.

If the pain is secondary to an injury, the physician must inquire about the mechanism of injury and any mechanical symptoms associated with it. The position of the joint at the time of traumatic force dictates which anatomic structures are at risk for injury. Therefore, it is important to allow the patient to describe the position of the knee and direction of forces of the injury. In addition, descriptions such as "locking," "popping," or "giving way" of the knee can aid in identifying the type of injury.[3]

After categorizing the knee pain in these broad categories, the clinician can better guide the interview and physical examination (described in later discussion) to narrow the differential and, ultimately, identify the underlying pathologic condition.

DIFFERENTIAL DIAGNOSIS FOR KNEE PAIN
History

When evaluating a patient with knee pain, it is important to consider the patient's complete medical history, including history of prior and recent injuries as well as chronic diseases, such as rheumatoid arthritis, lupus, fibromyalgia, obesity, gout, pseudogout, and degenerative joint disease.[3-8] Having a complete understanding of the patient can help the clinician understand and decipher the presenting symptoms (**Tables 1** and **2**).

Next, the physician should inquire about the pain, having the patient describe the onset, location, duration, severity, and quality of the pain. The onset may be acute or insidious, which can be a challenge to identify in the clinical setting, as many patients can present with acute exacerbations of a chronic problem. Asking about exacerbating and alleviating factors can help, particularly whether knee pain is worsened going up or down the stairs. The pain should then be localized (anterior, medial, lateral, or posterior knee) and characterized (dull, sharp, achy). Understanding the implication of the pain on the patient's function, mood, and lifestyle is also very important.

If an effusion is present, the timing of the effusion can help aid in the diagnosis of the injury. Rapid onset, within 2 hours, of a large effusion can suggest ACL rupture. Slower-onset effusion within 24 to 36 hours or recurrent knee effusion after activity is more consistent with meniscal injury.

Physical Examination

Inspection
A proper physical examination of the knee starts with a thorough inspection, which begins as the patient walks into the room, by observing their gait, balance, and use of cane or crutch.[3-7] Changes in gait may provide clues to injury patterns or the anatomic problem.

If swelling is present, it is important to distinguish effusion from other soft tissue swelling. Effusions may be large, tense, and easy to see, whereas others may be smaller and only detectable with careful palpation. Soft tissue swelling can also result in a swollen knee. Skin changes, such as ecchymosis, erythema, and abrasions, can help determine the cause of the swelling.

Palpation
After inspection, the knee joint must be palpated. Palpation is best performed when the knee is flexed to 90° as the patient is sitting on the examination table. A systematic approach to palpation will result in a complete and thorough examination. It is best to always start by examining the "good" knee first.

Table 1
Acute knee pain

Knee Pathologic Condition	History	Physical Examination
Anterior cruciate ligament tear	Common in young people who play sports associated with pivoting, decelerating, and jumping Audible "pop" followed by rapid joint swelling (1–2 h)	Lachman test Anterior drawer test Lateral pivot shift Swelling of the knee
Posterior cruciate ligament tear	Direct blow to the anterior aspect of the proximal tibia on a flexed knee with the ankle in plantarflexion Often occurs as dashboard injuries during motor vehicle accidents No "popping" sensation, minimal pain	Posterior sag sign Posterior drawer test Quadriceps active test Minimal swelling
Medial collateral ligament tear	Direct lateral force to the knee or noncontact injuries (common in skiing)	Valgus stress test Laxity of the joint
Lateral collateral ligament tear	Direct medial force to the knee	Varus stress test Laxity of the joint Often occurs in conjunction with other ligamentous tears, so must do a thorough examination
Meniscal tears	Occurs in younger individuals, mostly secondary to trauma Most common mechanism of injury is a twisting injury on a semiflexed limb through a weight-bearing knee "Locking" and "catching" sensations	McMurray test Joint line tenderness on palpation
Frank knee fracture	Frank fractures are due to direct trauma to the knee	Point tenderness to palpation at the site of fratture Inability to bear weight Decreased range of motion
Crystal arthropathy	Acute unilateral knee pain and swelling not related to trauma or activities Symptoms typically occur at night Typical joints: big toe, ankles, knees, elbows, wrists, fingers	Local erythema, warmth, joint pain, and effusion Reduced range of motion

Septic arthritis	Acute unilateral knee pain and swelling not related to trauma or activities Triad on presentation: fever + pain + impaired range of motion May present similarly to crystal arthropathy, but this is a medical emergency, so the two must be differentiated with joint aspiration and fluid analysis	Erythema, warmth, joint pain, and effusion Reduced range of motion
Osteoarthritis	Acute or chronic unilateral knee pain and swelling that may or may not be related to activities	Erythema, warmth, joint pain, crepitus, bony deformity, and effusion Reduced range of motion
Popliteal (Baker) cyst rupture	Posterior knee pain, knee stiffness, and swelling or a mass behind the knee (especially with the knee in extension) Discomfort with prolonged standing and with hyperflexion of the knee	Medial popliteal mass that is most prominent with the patient standing Swelling softens or disappears upon knee flexion to 45°

Table 2
Chronic knee pain

Knee Pathologic Condition	History	Physical Examination
Patellofemoral pain syndrome	Anterior knee pain that is aggravated by activities that increase patellofemoral compressive forces: ascending/ descending stairs, sitting with knees bent, kneeling, and squatting	Patellofemoral grinding test Apprehension test Tenderness to palpation of the patella
Stress fracture	Stress fractures are often a result of overuse Athletes often report an increase in training volume or intensity. Eventually pain worsens and may occur with rest	Point tenderness to palpation at the site of fracture Local swelling Pain increases with impact from running or jumping
Osteoarthritis	Use-related pain that is relieved by rest Pain begins as intermittent with use during high-impact activities, then may progress to pain with day-to-day activities Pain is often bilateral	Swelling and joint deformity may be present Crepitus and reduced range of motion
Pes anserine bursitis	Mild/moderate knee pain when arising from seated position or climbing stairs Worse at night Subjective complaints of muscle weakness and decreased range of motion of the knee joint	Tenderness to the proximal medial tibia 6 to 7 cm below the anteromedial joint line of the knee With knee flexion to 90°, tenderness to palpation along the medial tendinous structures of the pes anserine group as they travel to insert along the medial tibial region

The first thing to note on palpation is the skin temperature. At baseline, joints are typically cooler than their surrounding tissues because of their avascular nature. If the knee is the same temperature as the thigh or lateral calf, this may represent knee irritation and is not normal. The irritation may be due to joint effusion, meniscal injury, ligament tear, or fracture. If the knee is warmer than the thigh or lateral calf, this most commonly represents joint infection. Joint infection is typically accompanied by swelling and erythema of the joint. This pattern of joint warmth requires immediate evaluation with aspiration and analysis of synovial fluid because septic arthritis is a medical emergency.

The next thing to palpate is the medial and lateral joint lines. To do this, the examiner places their thumbs in the recesses inferolateral and inferomedial to the patella. Tenderness at the joint lines can reveal of the type damage that is present. Focal tenderness at a specific site typically indicates damage to a key structure in that location. Diffuse tenderness along a joint line, however, likely represents generalized irrigation of the synovial membrane, which may be secondary to a degenerative, inflammatory, or infectious process.

After palpation of the joint lines, the anterior and posterior knee should be palpated. Several structures are encountered with palpation of the anterior knee: tibial tuberosity, patellar tendon, patella, and quadriceps tendon. Tenderness to a specific structure in the anterior knee can aid in diagnosis of patellofemoral pain. In addition, palpation demonstrating point tenderness raises suspicion for the diagnosis of a fracture. In a normal knee, the only palpable item in the posterior knee should be the pulse of the popliteal artery. However, a sensation of pressure or fullness may be associated with joint effusion or a Baker cyst. If effusion is suspected, the physician can "milk the fluid" from the medial knee to the lateral aspect of the knee, and then compressing the lateral knee can result in the sudden appearance of a fluid bulge medial to the patella.

Range of motion
Determining the range of motion of the injured knee is crucial to making a diagnosis. Decreased range of motion may be secondary to swelling and pain; however, it can also aid in the diagnosis of a traumatic knee fracture. If there is crepitus on assessment of range of motion, osteoarthritis may be present. It is also critical to examine the hip joint, as hip injury or arthritis can cause referred pain to the knee. It is not uncommon to diagnose hip pathologic condition when a patient presents with knee pain, particularly in the elderly. Internal and external rotation of the hip joint is an important diagnostic maneuver with knee pain.

Special tests
Table 3 privides a list of condition-specific special tests.

Diagnostic Imaging

Plain radiograph
Plain radiographs of the knee are a commonly ordered diagnostic study to help in the evaluation of knee pain, yet they are often nondiagnostic of the most common causes for knee pain and only show fractures in 6% to 11% of cases of acute knee pain for which radiographs are obtained.[1] Most patients with acute knee pain have soft tissue injuries and, thus, plain film radiographs are not generally indicated and incur excess cost. One indication for plain radiograph imaging is if the history and physical examination lead to a concern for fracture. The Ottawa knee rules provide guidance as a clinical prediction tool to help clinicians reduce the number of unnecessary radiographs ordered after knee trauma without compromising patient care.

Patients must have one of the 4 Ottawa knee rules below to justify plain film imaging:

124   Farha et al

Table 3
Condition-specific special tests

Structure	Test	How to Perform Test	Evidence
Anterior cruciate ligament	Anterior drawer test	The patient is supine with their hip flexed to 45° and knee flexed to 90°. Examiner sits on the patient's foot with hands behind the proximal tibia and thumbs on the tibial plateau. Anterior force is applied to the proximal tibia Positive test: increased tibial displacement compared with the opposite side indicates ACL tear 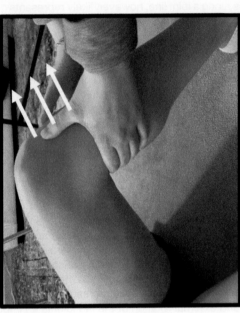	Sensitivity without anesthesia: 22.2%–41% Sensitivity with anesthesia: 79.6%–91% Specificity >97% Likelihood ratio: 3.8 (95% confidence interval [CI], 0.7–22.0) for a positive examination and 0.30 (95% CI, 0.05–1.50) for a negative examination
	Lachman test	Patient lies supine on the table with the involved extremity on the side of the examiner. With the patient's knee held between full extension and 15° of flexion, the femur is stabilized with 1 hand while firm pressure is applied to the posterior aspect of the proximal tibia in an attempt to translate it anteriorly Positive test: anterior translation of the tibia with "soft" endpoint indicates ACL rupture. This contrasts to a definite "hard" end point when the ACL is intact	Sensitivity: 80%–99% Specificity: 95% This test is the most sensitive and specific for diagnosing ACL tears

Likelihood ratio
25 (95% CI, 2.7–
651.0) for a positive
examination and 0.1
(CI 95%, 0.0–0.4) for
a negative examination

Sensitivity: 98.4%
Specificity: >98%

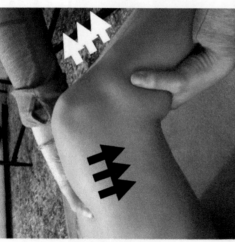

Lateral
pivot
shift

Patient rests on their back with the knee flexed to 45°. The examiner places a hand on the lateral aspect of the knee and pushes it medially, creating a valgus strain. At the same time, the examiner's other hand supports and pulls the foot laterally, extending the knee. The tibia and foot will begin to twist internally
Positive test: tibia will reduce at 30° flexion, and patients will typically express that they are done with the test. This indicates anterior subluxation of the tibia on the femur

(continued on next page)

Table 3
(continued)

Structure	Test	How to Perform Test	Evidence
Posterior cruciate ligament	Posterior sag sign	Patient lies supine with the hip flexed to 45° and the knee flexed to 90°. In this position, the tibia "rocks back" or sags back on the femur if the PCL is torn. Normally, the medial tibial plateau extends 1 cm anteriorly beyond the femoral condyle when the knee is flexed to 90°. If this step off is lost, it is considered positive for a PCL tear Positive test: tibia "rocks back" or sags back on the femur when positioned as stated above or loss of the "step off" between the medial tibial plateau and femoral condyle indicate a PCL tear	Sensitivity: 79% Specificity: 100%
	Posterior drawer test	Patient is supine with their hip flexed to 45° and knee flexed to 90°. Examiner sits on the patient's foot with hands behind the proximal tibia and thumbs on the tibial plateau. Posterior force is applied to the proximal tibia Positive test: increased tibial displacement compared with the opposite side indicates PCL tear	Sensitivity: 90% Specificity: 99%
	Quadriceps active test	With the patient supine, the relaxed limb is supported with the knee flexed to 90°. Contract the quadriceps to shift the tibia without extending the knee. In a normal knee, the patellar ligament is oriented slightly posterior and contraction of the quadriceps does not result in anterior shift of the tibia Positive test: tibia sags into posterior subluxation, and the patellar ligament is directed anteriorly in a PCL rupture	Sensitivity: 79% Specificity: 90%

| Medial collateral ligament | Valgus stress test | Patient is supine on the examination table with slight abduction of the hip and knee flexed to 30°. Examiner places 1 hand on the lateral aspect of the knee and grasps the ankle with the other hand. The examiner applies abduction (valgus) stress to the knee

Positive test: pain or clicking sensation when abduction is performed is positive for MCL laxity | | Sensitivity: 86%–96%
Specificity: not reported |
| Lateral collateral ligament | Varus stress test | Patient is supine on the examination table with slight abduction of the hip and knee flexed to 30°. Examiner places 1 hand on the lateral aspect of the knee and grasps the ankle with the other hand. The examiner applies adduction (varus) stress to the knee
Positive test: pain or clicking sensation when abduction is performed is positive for LCL laxity | | Sensitivity: 25%
Specificity: not reported |

(continued on next page)

Table 3
(continued)

Structure	Test	How to Perform Test	Evidence
Patellofemoral injuries	Patellofemoral grinding test	Clasp the patella with the thumb and index finger of each hand with the remainder of the fingers resting against the thigh and leg. When the patient lies with the leg relaxed and extended, the patella is pressed against the medial and lateral femoral condyles. Examiner moves the patella in an up-and-down fashion Positive test: pain with movement of the patella indicates patellofemoral dysfunction	No studies regarding sensitivity and specificity. This test is recommended against because it can cause pain in even asymptomatic subjects
	Apprehension test	Physician presses on the medial aspect of the patella with both thumbs, moving it laterally, while the knee is flexed to 30° with the quadriceps relaxed Positive test: when the patella approaches maximal displacement, the patient becomes uncomfortable and apprehensive, straightening the knee and moving the patella back to center. This is positive for patellar dislocation	Sensitivity: 39% Specificity: not reported
Meniscal injuries	McMurray test	Patient lies flat with the knee fully flexed until the heel approaches the buttock. The heel is held by the examiner's hand. The leg is then rotated on the thigh with the knee still in full flexion. By external rotation of the leg, the internal cartilage is tested, and by internal rotation of the leg, the external cartilage is tested Positive test: during this movement, the posterior section of the cartilage is rotated with the head of the tibia and, if any part of the cartilage or posterior section is loose, this movement produces an appreciable snap in the joint. This snap indicates meniscal injury	Sensitivity: 16%–58% Specificity: 77%–98% This test should not be overly emphasized when it is negative, given its low diagnostic sensitivity Likelihood ratio 1.3 (95% CI, 0.9–1.7) for a positive examination and 0.8 (95% CI, 0.6–1.1) for a negative examination

1. Age $\geq$55 years.
2. Isolated patellar tenderness or tenderness at the head of the fibula.
3. Inability to flex the knee 90°.
4. Inability to bear weight (4 steps) immediately after the injury and in the emergency department.

Although the Ottawa knee rules are sensitive, they have poor specificity. For this reason, only 3% of patients seen in primary care clinics who meet at least 1 criterion is ultimately diagnosed with a fracture. Not only do the Ottawa knee rules have flaws, but plain radiography itself is also not a perfect test. The sensitivity of knee radiographs ranges from 85% to 100%, and the specificity ranges from 88% to 92% for detecting fractures. Thus, 3 out of 1000 patients who meet the Ottawa knee rule criteria and have a negative radiograph will actually have a fracture.[1] In addition, patients who do not get knee films because of adherence with the Ottawa knee rules have a small risk of having a fracture. Thus, it is important for physicians to closely follow their patients with unexplained knee pain if something significant has been missed owing to poor imaging or lack of imaging.[9]

For chronic knee pain, plain standing knee radiography is the simplest, least expensive, and most used imaging modality for assessing for osteoarthritis. It helps visualize osteophytes, subchondral sclerosis, and cysts that may be present in the joint. It can also be used to grade the severity of the osteoarthritis using grading scales, such as the Kellgren and Lawrence grading system.[10]

MRI

The sensitivity of MRI is 75% to 87%, and the specificity is 80% to 93% for detecting meniscal, PCL, and ACL tears. However, the diagnostic accuracy of the physical examination is quite good, so MRI adds only marginal value when determining if a patient should be referred to an orthopedic surgeon. Thus, physicians should make the decision to refer based on their history and physical examination alone; the need for further diagnostic imaging can be determined by the surgeon.[11]

Ultrasound

Ultrasound is a useful tool in detecting knee effusions. Moderate- to large-volume effusions (20 mL +) are detectable on physical examination; however, smaller effusions can be missed. Ultrasound is approximately 100% sensitive and specific for detecting knee effusions, which is useful for detection of small effusions (5–10 mL) that are difficult to detect on physical examination. Effusions should be further evaluated with a complete history. Unexplained joint effusions always require arthrocentesis to rule out crystalline arthropathies, hemarthrosis, and infectious causes.[12]

In addition, ultrasound is a reliable, noninvasive method for detecting common disorders involving the tendons, ligaments, muscles, menisci, synovium, cartilage, and soft tissues of the knee joint. It can be used for grading osteoarthritis, as it helps identify inflammatory and structural abnormalities without contrast administration or exposure to radiation. In osteoarthritis, the main advantage of ultrasound over conventional radiography is the ability to detect synovial pathologic condition (hypertrophy, increased vascularity, presence of synovial fluid). In experienced hands, ultrasonography can play an important role in the assessment of pathologic conditions involving the knee joint.[13–15]

Management

Management of knee pain in the primary care clinic depends on a good history taking and physical examination in order to make an accurate diagnosis. The most important thing to determine is if the patient has an emergent condition, such as hemarthrosis and septic arthritis. Patients presenting with symptoms suggestive of one of these emergencies need be sent for urgent evaluation.

Lower-acuity causes of knee pain, such as Baker cysts and anserine bursitis, can be managed in the primary care clinic. Baker cysts are typically treated by addressing the underlying intraarticular inflammatory or degenerative processes. In patients with painful Baker cysts who want immediate, temporary relief, cyst aspiration followed by glucocorticoid injections is a low-risk and successful treatment.[16] Anserine bursitis can be managed conservatively with rest, ice, and short-term nonsteroidal anti-inflammatory drug (NSAID) use. In addition, in the setting of obesity, weight loss and strengthening of the quadriceps muscles can result in long-term resolution of symptoms.[8]

Typically, meniscal and ligamentous injuries should be referred to an orthopedic surgeon if mechanical symptoms are present (locking or catching). If the injury is minor, it can be managed by the primary care physician. The first-line therapy for these injuries is physical therapy and a structured exercise program. NSAIDs may provide short-term relief, but the risk of NSAIDs should always be considered and conveyed to the patient before initiating therapy. Finally, short-term use of a knee immobilizer may be beneficial immediately after an injury in order to protect the knee and maintain joint stability and support.[17]

More commonly, knee pain managed in the primary care clinic is due to osteoarthritis. In later discussion, the authors focus on the evidence-based approach to the management of knee pain resulting from osteoarthritis.

Weight loss
Among overweight and obese adults with osteoarthritis, diet and exercise resulting in weight loss of $\geq 10\%$ has been proven to result in less inflammation, less pain, better function, faster walking speed, and better physical health-related quality of life.[17–19]

Physical therapy/aquatic therapy
Physical therapy has proven to be useful in decreasing pain and increasing mobility in patients with osteoarthritis of the knee. Clinical physical therapy programs offer the benefits of on-site direction and availability of sophisticated equipment. Various studies have shown that physical therapy, including strengthening and aerobic exercises, can contribute to program adherence and overall better outcomes, including less pain and joint stiffness, greater physical function, and improvement in quality of life. In a randomized controlled trial, about 72% and 75% of participants reported improvements in pain and function, respectively, compared with only 17% (each) for control participants without therapy.[20]

One specific therapy that has been shown to be beneficial in patients with knee osteoarthritis is aquatic therapy, which involves exercise in water that is heated to about 32 to 36°C. A Cochrane review of aquatic therapy recommends that aquatic exercise be considered as the first part of an exercise therapy program to get particularly disabled patients introduced to training, as it is low-impact and showed positive effects on patients with knee osteoarthritis.[14]

Acetaminophen and nonsteroidal anti-inflammatory drugs
Acetaminophen and NSAIDs are first-line pharmacotherapy for osteoarthritis. Randomized controlled trials have shown acetaminophen to be as effective as ibuprofen. Given that acetaminophen has fewer adverse events than NSAIDs, it should be the first drug used to treat chronic knee pain. Extended-release acetaminophen (1300 mg 3 times daily) has been shown effective for treating knee pain secondary

to osteoarthritis.[21] In addition, a higher dose of ibuprofen (2400 mg per day) was not superior to a lower dose of ibuprofen (1200 mg per day) for pain relief or improvement of function, so if NSAIDs are used, a high dose is not necessary. Renal dose adjustments should be considered when applicable.[22,23]

Topical nonsteroidal anti-inflammatory drugs
Topical NSAIDs are often used for analgesia in lieu of oral NSAIDs, given the adverse risks associated with the oral form. They have been shown to be effective in reducing pain owing to chronic musculoskeletal conditions. The best data have been for topical diclofenac in osteoarthritis, where the number needed to treat for at least 50% pain relief over 8 to 12 weeks compared with placebo was 6.4 for the solution and 11 for the gel formulation. In addition, direct comparison of topical and oral NSAIDs has not shown any differences in efficacy.[24]

Duloxetine and gabapentin
Both duloxetine and gabapentin are often used in management of knee pain from osteoarthritis. One randomized clinical trial measured pain and functional status across 3 groups: patients received either gabapentin, duloxetine, or acetaminophen. It should be noted that duloxetine takes effect in the first weeks of initiation of therapy, whereas gabapentin takes full effect by the end of the third month of therapy. Both groups had a significant reduction in pain and improvement in functional status when compared with the acetaminophen group.[25]

Intraarticular injections
Intraarticular knee injections are often used for symptomatic relief while patients are waiting to get knee replacements. Two common intraarticular injections are glucocorticoid injections and hyaluronic acid injections. Glucocorticoid injections can be used to reduce pain by about 20% in the short term (1 to 3 weeks) in patients with osteoarthritis of the knee; however, no improvement has been seen at longer intervals. In addition, The American College of Rheumatology recommends that intraarticular corticosteroid injections be administered no more often than every 3 months for patients with osteoarthritis whose symptoms are not controlled with full-dose acetaminophen.[26,27]

Hyaluronic acid is a natural glycosaminoglycan that acts as a lubricant and elastic shock absorber during joint movement. The utility of intraarticular hyaluronic acid injections is 2-fold: they can protect against worsening of osteoarthritis while also providing analgesic effect on the joint.

Both glucocorticoid and hyaluronic acid injections are quite safe and provide similar benefit for improvement of knee function. The main difference between the 2 injections is that glucocorticoid injections are more effective at pain relief in the short term (up to 1 month), whereas hyaluronic acid is more effective for pain control for up to 6 months.[28]

Glucosamine and chondroitin sulfate
The dietary supplements glucosamine and chondroitin sulfate have been advocated by the media as safe and effective options for management of osteoarthritis symptoms. The data supporting this recommendation are of questionable quality. One randomized controlled trial of greater than 1500 patients revealed that glucosamine and chondroitin sulfate alone or in combination did not reduce pain effectively in patients with osteoarthritis of the knee. Currently, there is insufficient evidence to recommend use of these supplements.[29]

Arthroscopy

Arthroscopic intervention has been widely used in the past as a therapeutic intervention for patients with symptomatic osteoarthritis. However, significant evidence has shown no benefit to these procedures. One randomized controlled trial comparing arthroscopic lavage and debridement to those who underwent a placebo procedure showed no difference in outcomes. Another randomized trial compared outcomes in patients who underwent arthroscopic debridement and lavage in combination with medical and physical therapy to a group who had medical and physical therapy alone. At 2 years, there were no significant differences in the patients' pain, stiffness, and physical function. Thus, arthroscopic intervention is not recommended.[10,30]

Indications for referral

One of the most difficult decisions for a primary care physician is deciding when to refer a patient to a specialist for his/her knee pain. The recommendation is to refer for the following:

- Physical examination suggests ligament disruption
- Fracture of the knee is seen on imaging
- The patient has immediate marked swelling
- Aspiration reveals blood
- Aspiration reveals neutrophils or infection
- Physical examination reveals meniscal symptoms and mechanical locking
- Physical examination reveals meniscal symptoms and no mechanical locking AND patient has failed nonoperative therapy for 3 months
- If there is no improvement of acute knee pain within 7 to 10 days in certain cases

SUMMARY

Knee pain has a high prevalence in the general adult population and commonly presents in the primary care setting. There are many causes for knee pain, including systemic diseases, acute trauma, and degenerative joint disease. A detailed and focused history and physical examination are invaluable in identifying the cause of knee pain to further determine if imaging, physical therapy, specialty referral, or surgery is necessary. By following the above outlined systematic approach to evaluating knee pain, primary care physicians can make the correct diagnosis and formulate an appropriate therapeutic strategy for patients.

CASES

Case 1

A 73-year-old woman with a past medical history of hypertension, chronic obstructive pulmonary disease, and obesity comes into her primary care clinic complaining of pain in her left knee over the past 2 years that has gradually worsened. She does not have any history of knee trauma or injury. The pain used to only be present when she would walk her dog, but it now limits her daily activities, such as going up and down the stairs. The pain improves with acetaminophen and ibuprofen, but she is concerned about the repercussions of chronically taking these medications. What physical examination finding is most specific for this condition?

a. McMurray test
b. Crepitus with range of motion
c. Positive Lachman test
d. Laxity with valgus stress

Answer: B

This patient has a typical presentation of osteoarthritis. She has multiple risk factors, including advanced age, female gender, and obesity. Given her description of gradually worsening pain with activities and lack of inciting event, her picture is consistent with osteoarthritis. One of the hallmark physical examination findings of osteoarthritis is crepitus with range of motion.

McMurray test is positive in meniscal injuries. Meniscal injuries typically are a sequela of trauma and result in pain and swelling of the knee. Although only minor traumas can result in meniscal tears in older adults, this patient's story is more consistent with osteoarthritis than meniscal injury.

Positive Lachman test would be consistent with an ACL injury. Typically, ACL injuries are a result of trauma. The classic presentation is someone who has an injury while playing sports (jumping, sudden stopping, decelerating), hears a "pop," and then has swelling within 1 to 2 hours.

Laxity with valgus stress would be consistent with a MCL tear; this would typically be the result of traumatic blow to the lateral knee.

Case 2

A 56-year-old man with a past medical history of depression and gastroesophageal reflux disease presents at urgent care because of right knee pain after falling while playing basketball with his daughter earlier this morning. He is walking with crutches because of an inability to bear weight. On physical examination, soft tissue swelling and ecchymosis are noted. He has tenderness to palpation of the head of the proximal fibula. He has full range of motion, although movement is painful. What is the next best step for the management of this man's knee pain?

a. MRI
b. Consult to orthopedic surgery
c. Plain film radiograph
d. Conservative management and follow up in 4 weeks

Answer: C

This man meets three of the criteria of the Ottawa knee rules, a guide to help identify individuals at risk of having a knee fracture who would benefit from plain film imaging. The rules are as follows:

1. Age $\geq$55 years
2. Isolated patellar tenderness or tenderness at the head of the fibula
3. Inability to flex the knee 90°
4. Inability to bear weight (4 steps) immediately after the injury and in the emergency department

This patient is $\geq$55 years old, has tenderness at the head of the fibula, and is unable to bear weight in the urgent care, thus, meeting three of the criteria. Therefore, he would benefit from plain film imaging of his knee, as he is at a high risk of having a fracture.

MRI is best for seeing ligamentous and meniscal injuries, but in a patient with a high likelihood of fracture, plain film radiograph is the next best step given its low cost and high yield. A consult to orthopedic surgery may be required in a patient with trauma to the knee, but it is best to obtain plain film imaging before determining the need for the consult.

Case 3

A 23-year-old woman presents to her primary care physician because of left knee pain after being kicked during soccer practice yesterday. She describes being kicked in the anterior knee and then hearing an audible "pop." Since then, she notes some increased fullness in her knee and bruising on the front of her knee. The physician performs a physical examination maneuver whereby the patient is laying on her back with her left knee flexed to 90°; the examiner then pushes the tibia posteriorly. What is this examination maneuver called and what indicates a positive test?

a. Lachman test; pain
b. Lachman test; lack of a distinct endpoint
c. Posterior drawer test; pain
d. Posterior drawer test; laxity

Answer: B
This young woman presents with likely injury to her PCL. The classic presentation for PCL injury is an anterior blow to the knee, resulting in a popping sound, pain, and fullness in the knee. The physical examination maneuver described is the posterior drawer test, which is positive if the PCL is injured, resulting in laxity when compared with the other side. Pain may be present as well, but is not specific to this test and, thus, does not constitute a positive test.

The Lachman test is used to identify ACL injuries. This test is performed by placing the knee in 30° of flexion and then stabilizing the distal femur with 1 hand while pulling the proximal tibia anteriorly with the other hand. A normal ACL results in a distinct endpoint; a positive test is present when there lacks a distinct endpoint. This maneuver may also be associated with pain, but that does not necessitate a positive test.

CLINICS CARE POINTS

- Identifying traumatic versus atraumatic knee pain is a critical initial step in evaluating etiology of knee pain.
- There are clear indications for plain radiography of the knee in the setting of acute knee injuries, as defined by the Ottawa Knee Rules.
- One of the most common causes of chronic, atraumatic knee pain seen in primary care clinics is osteoarthritis.
- The physical examination is an important part of evaluation of knee pain, and several special maneuvers can be used to identify the etiology of knee pain.
- Initial management of osteoarthritic knee pain involves lifestyle modifications. Weight loss of > 10% has been proven to result in less inflammation, less pain, better function, faster walking speed, and better physical health-related quality of life. Aquatic therapy is recommended as an initial exercise therapy program, as it is low-impact and has shown positive effects on patients with osteoarthritis of the knee.
- Initial pharmacologic management for osteoarthritic knee pain involves use of acetaminophen and nonsteroidal anti-inflammatory drugs. A higher dose of ibuprofen (2400 mg per day) was not superior to a lower dose of ibuprofen (1200 mg per day) for pain relief or improvement of function.

DISCLOSURE

The authors have no conflicts of interest to disclose.

REFERENCES

1. Jackson JL, O'Malley PG, Kroenke K. Evaluation of acute knee pain in primary care. Ann Intern Med 2003;139(7):575–88.
2. Solomon DH, Simel DL, Bates DW, et al. The rational clinical examination. Does this patient have a torn meniscus or ligament of the knee? Value of the physical examination. JAMA 2001;286(13):1610–20.
3. Calmbach WL, Hutchens M. Evaluation of patients presenting with knee pain: part I. History, physical examination, radiographs, and laboratory tests. Am Fam Physician 2003;68:907–12.
4. Rossi R, Dettoni F, Bruzzone M, et al. Clinical examination of the knee: know your tools for diagnosis of knee injuries. Sports Med Arthrosc Rehabil Ther Technol 2011;3:25.
5. Malanga GA, Andrus S, Nadler SF, et al. Physical examination of the knee: a review of the original test description and scientific validity of common orthopedic tests. Arch Phys Med Rehabil 2003;84(4):592–603.
6. Haim A, Pritsch T, Yosepov L, et al. Anterior cruciate ligament injuries. Harefuah 2006;145(3):208–14, 244–5.
7. Schulz MS, Russe K, Weiler A, et al. Epidemiology of posterior cruciate ligament injuries. Arch Orthop Trauma Surg 2003;123(4):186–91.
8. Mohseni M, Graham C. Pes anserine bursitis. In: StatPearls [Internet]. Treasure Island (FL): StatPearls Publishing; 2020.
9. Yao K, Haque T. The Ottawa knee rules - a useful clinical decision tool. Aust Fam Physician 2012;41(4):223–4.
10. Moseley JB, O'Malley K, Petersen NJ, et al. A controlled trial of arthroscopic surgery for osteoarthritis of the knee. N Engl J Med 2002;347:81–8.
11. Boeve BF, Davidson RA, Staab EV Jr. Magnetic resonance imaging in the evaluation of knee injuries. South Med J 1991;84(9):1123–7.
12. Zuber T. Knee joint aspiration and injection. Am Fam Physician 2002;55(8):1497–501.
13. Razek AA, Fouda NS, Elmetwaley N, et al. Sonography of the knee joint( ). J Ultrasound 2009;12(2):53–60.
14. Hayashi D, Roemer FW, Guermazi A. Imaging for osteoarthritis. Ann Phys Rehabil Med 2016;59:161–9.
15. Bartels EM, Lund H, Hagen KB, et al. Aquatic exercise for the treatment of knee and hip osteoarthritis. Cochrane Database Syst Rev 2007;(4):CD005523.
16. Herman AM, Marzo JM. Popliteal cysts: a current review. Orthopedics 2014;37(8):e678–84.
17. Jones BQ, Covey CJ, Sineath MH. Nonsurgical management of knee pain in adults. Am Fam Physician 2015;92:875–83.
18. Hochberg MC, Altman RD, April KT, et al. American College of Rheumatology 2012 recommendations for the use of nonpharmacologic and pharmacologic therapies in osteoarthritis of the hand, hip, and knee. Arthritis Care Res (Hoboken) 2012;64(4):465–74.
19. Messier SP, Mihalko SL, Legault C, et al. Effects of intensive diet and exercise on knee joint loads, inflammation, and clinical outcomes among overweight and obese adults with knee osteoarthritis: the IDEA randomized clinical trial. JAMA 2013;310(12):1263–73.
20. Bhatia D, Bejarano T, Novo M. Current interventions in the management of knee osteoarthritis. J Pharm Bioallied Sci 2013;5(1):30–8.

21. Prior MJ, Harrison DD, Frustaci ME. A randomized, double-blind, placebo-controlled 12 week trial of acetaminophen extended release for the treatment of signs and symptoms of osteoarthritis. Curr Med Res Opin 2014;30(11): 2377–87.
22. Bradley JD, Brandt KD, Katz BP, et al. Comparison of an antiinflammatory dose of ibuprofen, an analgesic dose of ibuprofen, and acetaminophen in the treatment of patients with osteoarthritis of the knee. N Engl J Med 1991;325(2):87–91.
23. Verkleij SP, Luijsterburg PA, Bohnen AM, et al. NSAIDs vs acetaminophen in knee and hip osteoarthritis: a systematic review regarding heterogeneity influencing the outcomes. Osteoarthritis Cartilage 2011;19(8):921–9.
24. Derry S, Moore RA, Rabbie R. Topical NSAIDs for chronic musculoskeletal pain in adults. Cochrane Database Syst Rev 2012;(9):CD007400.
25. Enteshari-Moghaddam A, Azami A, Isazadehfar K, et al. Efficacy of duloxetine and gabapentin in pain reduction in patients with knee osteoarthritis. Clin Rheumatol 2019;38:2873–80.
26. Bellamy N, Campbell J, Robinson V, et al. Intraarticular corticosteroid for treatment of osteoarthritis of the knee. Cochrane Database Syst Rev 2006;(2):CD005328.
27. Jones T, Kelsberg G, Safranek S. FPIN's clinical inquiries: intra-articular corticosteroid injections for osteoarthritis of the knee. Am Fam Physician 2014;90(2): 115–6.
28. He WW, Kuang MJ, Zhao J, et al. Efficacy and safety of intraarticular hyaluronic acid and corticosteroid for knee osteoarthritis: a meta-analysis. Int J Surg 2017; 39:95–103.
29. Clegg DO, Reda DJ, Harris CL, et al. Glucosamine, chondroitin sulfate, and the two in combination for painful knee osteoarthritis. N Engl J Med 2006;354: 795–808.
30. Kirkley A, Birmingham TB, Litchfield RB, et al. A randomized trial of arthroscopic surgery for osteoarthritis of the knee. N Engl J Med 2008;359:1097–107.

Approach to Fatigue
Best Practice

Jason C. Dukes, MD, MBA, M.Sc[a],*, Matthew Chakan, MD[b],
Aaron Mills, DO[c], Maurice Marcaurd, MD[d]

KEYWORDS

- Fatigue • Tiredness • Sleepiness • Chronic fatigue syndrome • Myalgic encephalitis
- Systemic exertion intolerance disease

KEY POINTS

- An estimated 5% to 10% of primary care visits are directly related to fatigue.
- Numerous diagnostic tools exist to assist with fatigue differentiation such as Epworth Sleepiness Scale, STOP-Bang questionnaire, Patient Health Questionnaire-9, and the Chalder Fatigue Scale.
- Performance of a battery of diagnostic tests is unlikely to assist with diagnosis, highlighting the importance of a patient-centered differential diagnosis through a comprehensive history of presenting illness, review of systems, and physical examination.
- Management of fatigue largely depends on identifying the presence of an underlying condition and treating it accordingly.
- Systemic exertion intolerance disease (formerly chronic fatigue syndrome or myalgic encephalitis) is diagnosed when a patient has fatigue for greater than 6 months, postexertional malaise, unrefreshing sleep, in addition to one of the following: cognitive impairment or orthostatic intolerance.

COMMON SYMPTOMS IN OUTPATIENT PRACTICE
Fatigue

Introduction
Fatigue is one of the most frequent presenting complaints to the primary care office. It is estimated that between 5% and 10% of all primary care visits are directly related to fatigue.[1,2] The overall estimation of fatigue in the general population is much higher with a wide range of prevalence from 7% to 45%.[3] The wide variation in prevalence

[a] Internal Medicine Department, Eastern Virginia Medical School, 825 Fairfax Avenue, Suite 565, Norfolk, VA 23507, USA; [b] Internal Medicine Department, Eastern Virginia Medical School, 825 Fairfax Avenue, Suite 481, Norfolk, VA 23507, USA; [c] Internal Medicine Department, Eastern Virginia Medical School, 825 Fairfax Avenue, Suite 483, Norfolk, VA 23507, USA; [d] Internal Medicine Department, Eastern Virginia Medical School, 825 Fairfax Avenue, Suite 572, Norfolk, VA 23507, USA
* Corresponding author.
E-mail address: dukesjc@evms.edu

Med Clin N Am 105 (2021) 137–148
https://doi.org/10.1016/j.mcna.2020.09.007
0025-7125/21/© 2020 Elsevier Inc. All rights reserved.

stems from inconsistent definitions of fatigue and lack of patient reporting. In the United States, fatigue is estimated to cost nearly $100 billion annually due to loss of productivity.[2] Although the complaint is commonplace, the underlying cause is oftentimes not ascertained due to the vague nature of the presenting symptoms. Its meaning can also be influenced by a patient's culture.[4] Owing to the very broad, and potentially fatal, differential diagnoses that can present as fatigue, a rational approach to diagnosis is critical. Performing a battery of diagnostic tests is unlikely to assist with diagnosis,[5,6] highlighting the importance of forming an appropriately prioritized patient-centered differential diagnosis through a comprehensive history of presenting illness, review of systems, and physical examination.[5,6]

Definitions: sleepiness versus fatigue

Although fatigue is a common complaint, it may be confused with sleepiness as patients often present with a vague complaint of being "tired" or "exhausted".[7] The interchangeability of the terms sleepiness and fatigue can lead clinicians down a diagnostic path that is rarely fruitful. Although it may seem apparent, the generally accepted definition of sleepiness is the increased likelihood of falling asleep.[8] This includes both inappropriate and appropriate times to fall asleep. In the primary care setting, the primary concern is with the increased likelihood of falling asleep at inappropriate times and is potentially better defined as excessive daytime sleepiness.[8]

By contrast, fatigue has an ambiguous definition and is generally described as a lack of energy, overwhelming feeling of exhaustion, and impaired cognitive or physical function.[8] Pigeon and colleagues[9] proposes that sleepiness should be defined as drowsiness, decreased alertness, or increased sleep propensity, whereas fatigue is described as weariness, weakness, or depleted energy. Whichever definition is used (**Table 1**), it is important to clarify whether the patient describes having sleepiness or fatigue. This can be done by asking direct and specific questions such as, "Do you often find yourself falling asleep during the day?" and "Do you find yourself unable to participate in activities due to quick exhaustion?". Generally, sleepiness will improve with activity whereas fatigue will remain or worsen, which can be another useful characteristic to differentiate between them.[7]

It is also important to define acute versus chronic fatigue as the differential possibilities greatly depend on the duration. Acute fatigue is defined as less than 1 month, whereas chronic fatigue is defined as greater than six months.[10] Prolonged fatigue is between 1 and 6 months.[10]

History

Acute fatigue is often attributable to a self-limited condition, whereas an underlying cause of chronic fatigue is often unidentified (**Fig. 1**).[11] Patients may improve over

Table 1
Definitions of sleepiness versus fatigue

Current Terms	Shen et al. Definitions	Pigeon et al. Definitions
Sleepiness	Increases propensity of falling asleep	Drowsiness, sleep propensity, and decreased alertness
Fatigue	Impaired physical or cognitive function, lack of energy, and overwhelming feeling of exhaustion	Weariness, weakness, depleted energy

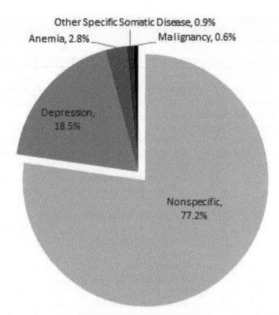

Fig. 1. Etiology of a primary or secondary complaint of fatigue in primary care patients.

the next several months and will have multiple follow-up visits in which to reassess for the presence of a missed worrisome diagnosis.[6,12]

Paramount to this evaluation is the disambiguation of the individualized meaning of fatigue through a careful history and comprehensive review of systems including quality, severity or impact, timing, aggravating or alleviating factors, and associated symptoms. Clarification of a single fatigue complaint can reveal aspects of sleepiness (91%), poor concentration (76%), difficulty completing an activity (63%), muscle weakness (56%), or muscle pain (51%).[13] This forms the basis of the differential diagnosis (**Table 2**).

A complaint of fatigue that is associated with a desire to sleep when at rest and improves with sleep or activity may represent an underlying sleep disorder (see **Table 2**). Taking a focused sleep history including sleep location, bedtime, evening medication or substance use, time to initiation, frequency and reason for awakenings, sleep duration, subjective sleep adequacy on awakening, bed-partner complaints such as snoring or movements, and recent changes with work or travel schedules. Completing the Epworth Sleepiness Scale (**Table 3**) or STOP-Bang Questionnaire (**Table 4**) may provide further information to clarify the diagnoses.

A complaint of fatigue that is associated with symptoms of a depressed mood, diminished interest or pleasure, feeling of worthlessness, poor concentration, or recurrent thoughts of death may represent major depressive disorder. Completing the Patient Health Questionnaire-9 (**Fig. 2**) may be elucidative.

A complaint of fatigue that is associated with difficulty completing activities requires further clarification of the types of activities attempted and specific reasons for incompletion. Patients may describe chest pain, palpitations, pedal edema, dyspnea on exertion, dizziness, or focal sensorimotor deficits. Eliciting specific symptoms may narrow the differential diagnosis and reveal a distinct investigational and management pathway. Specific consideration should also be given to reviewing the medication list and substance abuse history, as several substances are

Table 2
Differential diagnoses of secondary fatigue

Sleepiness	Poor Concentration	Difficulty Completing Activities	Muscle Pain
Insomnia	Attention deficit	Acute coronary syndrome	Epstein-Barr virus
Obstructive	disorder	Anemia	Fibromyalgia
sleep apnea	Anorexia/bulimia	Arrhythmia	Hepatitis C
Periodic limb	Bipolar depression	COPD	HIV
movement	Generalized anxiety	Cirrhosis	Hypothyroidism
disorder	disorder	Congestive heart failure	Hypogonadism
Poor sleep	Major depressive	Deconditioning	Inclusion body myositis
hygiene	disorder	Diabetes	Lyme
		End stage renal disease	Polymyalgia rheumatica
		Inflammatory bowel disease	Polymyositis
		Malignancy	Rheumatoid arthritis
		Medication adverse effect	Systemic lupus
		Multiple sclerosis	erythematosus
		Neuromuscular junction	
		disorders	
		Osteoarthritis	
		Polyneuropathy	
		Pregnancy	
		Pulmonary embolism	
		Pulmonary hypertension	
		Stroke	
		Substance use disorder	

commonly implicated. Special consideration should also be given to pregnancy in sexually active women of childbearing age, as fatigue is ubiquitously reported (97%) in the first trimester.[14]

A complaint of fatigue that is associated with muscle pain requires further clarification of the involved distribution, quality, radiation, severity, timing, aggravating or

Table 3
Epworth sleepiness scale

How Likely Are You to Doze Off or Fall Asleep in the Following Situations?			
			3 = High Chance
0 = No Chance 1 = Slight Chance 2 = Moderate Chance			Chance of Dozing
Sitting and reading	0	1	2 3
Watching television	0	1	2 3
Sitting inactive in a public place	0	1	2 3
As a passenger in a car for an hour without a break	0	1	2 3
Lying down to rest in the afternoon when circumstances permit	0	1	2 3
Sitting and talking to someone	0	1	2 3
Sitting quietly after a lunch without alcohol	0	1	2 3
In a car, while stopped for a few minutes in traffic	0	1	2 3
Interpretation			
Normal	EDS		High Levels of EDS
0-10	>10		>16

Abbreviation: EDS, excessive daytime sleepiness.

Table 4		
STOP-Bang questionnaire		
Questions	Yes	No
Do you snore?		
Do you often feel tired, fatigued, or sleepy during the day?		
Has anyone observed that you stop breathing during your sleep?		
Do you have high blood pressure?		
Is your BMI above 35?		
Are you older than 50 years of age?		
Is your neck circumference greater than 40 cm?		
Are you male?		
1 point for positive responses. 0-2 low risk, 3/4 intermediate risk, 5 or more high risk		

alleviating factors, and associated symptoms. Numerous infectious and non-infectious inflammatory conditions as well as endocrinopathies have been associated with fatigue (see **Table 2**). Patients may describe an acute onset after a febrile illness that could suggest an acute viral or bacterial infection, whereas a chronic duration could suggest a rheumatologic, endocrinologic, or occult viral or bacterial infection. Specific consideration should be given to assessing a patient's risk for acquiring occult infections through travel, substance abuse, and sexual histories.

Although hypothyroidism is frequently assessed in the absence of multisymptom hypothyroid syndrome, where fatigue or tiredness is the most frequently reported symptom (81%), hypothyroidism is less likely in the absence of at least one additional symptom.[6,15–17] The likelihood of diagnosing hypothyroidism increases with the number of associated symptoms as well as symptom progression over time.[15–17] Consider assessing additional symptoms such as deepening voice, hoarseness, decreased sweating, constipation, hair loss, slowed thinking, muscle cramps, cold intolerance, and weight gain.[15–17]

In addition to evaluating the characteristics of fatigue, an assessment of negative prognostic features is also warranted. A delayed recovery can be associated with a patient expectation of chronicity, higher fatigue severity, and lack of social support.[18]

Diagnostic tools
There are several patient-centered tools that can be used to help differentiate the causes of fatigue. Some of these include the Epworth Sleepiness Scale, the STOP-Bang questionnaire, and the Patient Health Questionnaire-9 (PHQ9).

The Epworth Sleepiness Scale is a reliable tool that can help differentiate sleepiness and fatigue.[19] This tool (see **Table 3**) is used to quantify a patient's sleepiness, with higher scores suggesting sleepiness as a cause.[19]

The STOP-Bang questionnaire (see **Table 4**) can help stratify the risk of sleep apnea, with a higher score indicating greater risk.[19,20] Sleep apnea is a relatively common condition that is often underdiagnosed.

The PHQ9 (see **Fig. 2**) is used to evaluate for depression which is common and could represent an underlying cause for fatigue.[21,22] Patients who are found to have depression should be treated and have their PHQ9 scores followed for improvement.

Chalder Fatigue Scale (**Table 5**) is a tool used to gauge severity of fatigue.[23] There are several other questionnaires available for determining severity of fatigue, especially if related to underlying chronic medical problems.[23]

PATIENT HEALTH QUESTIONNAIRE (PHQ-9)

NAME:_____   DATE:_____

Over the last 2 weeks, how often have you been
bothered by any of the following problems?
(use "✓" to indicate your answer)

	Not at all	Several days	More than half the days	Nearly every day
1. Little interest or pleasure in doing things	0	1	2	3
2. Feeling down, depressed, or hopeless	0	1	2	3
3. Trouble falling or staying asleep, or sleeping too much	0	1	2	3
4. Feeling tired or having little energy	0	1	2	3
5. Poor appetite or overeating	0	1	2	3
6. Feeling bad about yourself—or that you are a failure or have let yourself or your family down	0	1	2	3
7. Trouble concentrating on things, such as reading the newspaper or watching television	0	1	2	3
8. Moving or speaking so slowly that other people could have noticed. Or the opposite — being so fidgety or restless that you have been moving around a lot more than usual	0	1	2	3
9. Thoughts that you would be better off dead, or of hurting yourself	0	1	2	3

add columns   [   ] + [   ] + [   ]

(Healthcare professional: For interpretation of TOTAL,   TOTAL: [   ]
please refer to accompanying scoring card).

10. If you checked off any problems, how difficult have these problems made it for you to do your work, take care of things at home, or get along with other people?	Not difficult at all _____
	Somewhat difficult _____
	Very difficult _____
	Extremely difficult _____

Fig. 2. Patient health Questionnaire-9. (Courtesy of Pfitzer Inc, New York, NY.)

Table 5
Chalder fatigue scale

Questions	Less than Usual	No More than Usual	More than Usual	Much More than Usual
Do you have problems with tiredness?				
Do you need more rest?				
Do you feel sleepy or drowsy?				
Do you have problems starting things?				
Do you lack energy?				
Do you have less strength in your muscles?				
Do you feel weak?				
Do you have difficulties concentrating?				
Do you make slips of the tongue when speaking?				
Do you find it more difficult to find the right word?				
	Better than usual	No worse than usual	Worse than usual	Much worse than usual
How is your memory?				

Scoring is 0-3 with max sore 33—higher the score indicates more severe fatigue

These tools are only some of the many that are available to the medical community to help in properly diagnosing patients.

Evaluation and management

Once sleepiness and fatigue have been separated, evaluation aims to determine if the patient is suffering from primary or secondary fatigue. Secondary fatigue is seen in patients who have an underlying medical condition causing their symptom.[24] This can be done primarily with a thorough history and physical looking for signs of underlying medical problems as discussed earlier.

Laboratory testing without a positive finding on history and physical is rarely helpful.[25] Typically laboratory testing will show minor abnormalities that do not help in a diagnosis.[25] However, if the history or physical suggests a high pre-test probability for an underlying medical cause or potential red flags, further testing is warranted (**Table 6**).

Proper sleep is important to discuss with patients to ensure that sleepiness is not contributing to the fatigue as they are often interlinked and can be difficult to discern.[26] Evaluating patients in a stepwise fashion assists in differentiating the diagnosis without unnecessary testing (**Fig. 3**). Management of fatigue largely depends on identifying the presence of an underlying condition and treating it accordingly (**Table 7**).

Systemic exertion intolerance disease

Fatigue can be a sequela of an underlying medical disease or exists as a primary condition. Previously, primary fatigue was referred to as chronic fatigue syndrome (CFS)

Table 6
Potential red flags

History/Physical Finding	Diagnosis	Test(s) to Consider
Anticoagulation use	Anemia	CBC
Dyspnea on exertion	Acute myocardial infarction, CHF	ECG, echocardiogram
Insulin use	Hypoglycemia	Glucose monitoring
Neurologic deficit	Stroke	CT head
Night sweats	Tuberculosis	PPD
Oliguria	AKI, CKD, ESRD	Chemistry panel
Palpitations	Cardiac arrhythmia	ECG, Holter monitor
Shortness of breath, tachycardia	Pulmonary embolism	Chest CT A, d-dimer

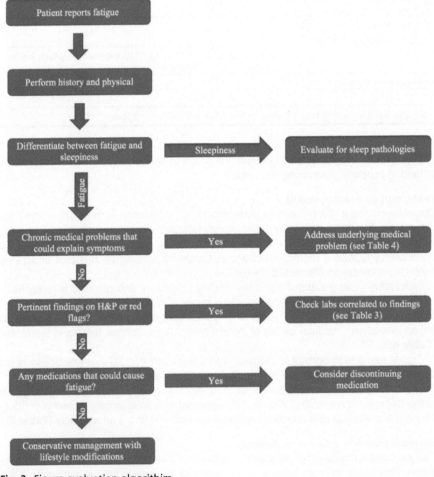

Fig. 3. Figure evaluation algorithim.

Table 7 **Indications for testing**		
Disease	**Clinical Finding**	**Test(s) to Consider**
Anemia	Pallor, menorrhagia	Complete blood count
Arrythmia	Exercise intolerance, palpitations	ECG
Diabetes	Polyuria, polydipsia	Hemoglobin A1C
CHF	Edema, decreased exercise tolerance	BNP
COPD	Shortness of breath, barrel chest	Spirometry
Electrolyte abnormalities	Muscle pains and spasms	Chemistry panel
Hepatitis	Hepatomegaly, alcohol use	Liver function test
HIV	Weight loss, sexual activity, flu-like symptoms	HIV antibody testing
Hypothyroid	Cold, dry skin, weight gain	TSH
PMR	Muscle pain/stiffness proximally	Sedimentation rate
Pregnant	Female, childbearing age, recent unprotected sex, amenorrhea	Urine pregnancy test
Viral infection	Acute onset, combined with viral symptoms	Influenza, respiratory viral panel

This is a brief overview of more common possibilities - further testing should be done if warranted by findings in the history and physical.

or myalgic encephalitis (ME). CFS and ME were initially thought of as two distinct entities with separate diagnostic criteria. This made it challenging to diagnose and manage CFS and ME.

In addition to the confusion created by the striking similarities between CFS and ME, a stigma is associated with these terms. Unfortunately, there is skepticism among medical providers about the debilitating nature of CFS and ME. Patients have been told that this is a psychogenic illness, although systemic features are now known to exist. Part of the misinformation is based in large part on the lack of provider education. Less than a third of medical schools have curriculum dedicated to CFS and ME.[27]

With this in mind, the Institute of Medicine (now the National Academy of Medicine) convened a committee to examine the existing diagnostic criteria of both CFS and ME to establish unified and streamlined criteria. In 2015, the National Academy of Medicine released a comprehensive report which revised criteria (**Box 1**) and changed CFS and ME to systemic exertion intolerance disease (SEID).[28]

It is estimated that anywhere between 836,000 and 2.5 million Americans have SEID.[29] Between 84% and 91% of patients are undiagnosed and up to 29% have reported taking longer than 5 years to diagnose.[29,30] SEID causes significant harm to the individual and surrounding community. Direct and indirect economic costs to society have been quoted at $24 billion annually.[31]

Diagnostic criteria of SEID[28] The pathogenesis of this disorder remains unknown. In many cases, symptoms are associated with a preceding infection or other event.[32] The theory of central sensitization is considered a potential cause of SEID, but remains an area of ongoing research. In 2019, a systematic review was performed exploring the role of cytokines in SEID to determine if there was a significant difference in cytokine levels between those with SEID versus the general population. Fifteen observational case-control studies were included in the review. The findings of this review were inconclusive regarding the role of cytokines in SEID.[33]

> **Box 1**
> **Diagnostic criteria of SEID**
>
> Presence of all of the following:
> - A substantial reduction or impairment in the ability to engage in preillness levels of occupational, educational, social or personal activities that persists for more than 6 months and is accompanied by fatigue, which is often profound, is of new or definite onset (not lifelong), is not the result of ongoing excessive exertion, and is not substantially alleviated by rest.
> - Postexertional malaise[a]
> - Unrefreshing sleep[a]
>
> Presence of at least one of the following manifestations is also required:
> - Cognitive impairment[a]
> - Orthostatic intolerance (symptoms such as lightheadedness, dizziness, and headache that are exacerbated with erect posture and improve when recumbent)
>
> [a] Frequency and severity of symptoms should be assessed. The diagnosis of SEID should be questioned if patients do not have these symptoms at least half of the time with moderate, substantial, or severe intensity.
>
> *Data from* IOM (Institute of Medicine). Beyond Myalgic Encephalomyelitis/Chronic Fatigue Syndrome: Redefining an Illness. Washington (DC): National Academies Press (US); 2015 Feb 10.

Unfortunately, there are no FDA-approved medications for SEID. Pharmacotherapy should be reserved for treating comorbid conditions such as depression. Remaining active is paramount to improve fatigue and overall functioning, but exercise therapy must be individualized.[34] In addition, several studies suggest that cognitive behavioral therapy is beneficial in some patients.[35] Before starting an intervention, fatigue severity should be determined using a scoring questionnaire.[23] This can be repeated as different therapies are trialed to monitor the patient's improvement with each therapy.[23] Stimulants are not recommended as they rarely help symptoms and are associated with several side effects.[24] Providers should schedule frequent office visits for longitudinal reassessment. Because there is no established treatment of SEID, it is important that providers reassure patients that their symptoms are real. A healthy patient-provider relationship is critical to successfully managing SEID.

CLINICS CARE POINTS

- It important to distinguish between sleepiness and fatigue. Generally, sleepiness will improve with activity whereas fatigue will remain or worsen.[7]
- Depression was diagnosed in 18.5% of patients with a primary or secondary complaint of fatigue in primary care patients.[11]
- Hypothyroidism is frequently assessed in the evaluation of fatigue. In the absence of additional symptoms (e.g. cold intolerance, weight gain, constipation), hypothyroidism is less likely.[15–17]
- There is significant underdiagnosis of systemic exertion intolerance disease (SEID). In up 29% of patients with SEID, diagnosis took longer than five years.[29,30]
- Stimulants are not recommended to treat SEID.[24]

DISCLOSURE

The authors have nothing to disclose.

REFERENCES

1. Nicholson K, Stewart M, Thind A. Examining the symptom of fatigue in primary care: a comparative study using electronic medical records. J Innov Health Inform 2015;22(1):235–43.
2. Ricci JA, Chee E, Lorandeau AL, et al. Fatigue in the U.S. Workforce: Prevalence and Implications for Lost Productive Work Time. J Occup Environ Med 2007; 49(1):1–10.
3. Junghaenel DU, Christodoulou C, Lai J-S, et al. Demographic correlates of fatigue in the US general population: Results from the patient-reported outcomes measurement information system (PROMIS) initiative. J Psychosom Res 2011; 71(3):117–23.
4. Cho HJ, Bhugra D, Wessely S. 'Physical or psychological?'– a comparative study of causal attribution for chronic fatigue in Brazilian and British primary care patients. Acta Psychiatr Scand 2008;118(1):34–41.
5. Lane TJ, Matthews DA, Manu P. The Low Yield of Physical Examinations and Laboratory Investigations of Patients with Chronic Fatigue. Am J Med Sci 1990; 299(5):313–8.
6. Kitai E, Blumberg G, Levy D, et al. Fatigue as a first-time presenting symptom: management by family doctors and one year follow-up. Isr Med Assoc J 2012; 14:555–9.
7. Shen J, Botly LCP, Chung SA, et al. Fatigue and shift work. J Sleep Res 2006; 15(1):1–5.
8. Shen J, Barbera J, Shapiro CM. Distinguishing sleepiness and fatigue: focus on definition and measurement. Sleep Med Rev 2005;10(1):63–76.
9. Pigeon WR, Sateia MJ, Ferguson RJ. Distinguishing between excessive daytime sleepiness and fatigue. J Psychosom Res 2003;54(1):61–9.
10. Son CG. Differential diagnosis between "chronic fatigue" and "chronic fatigue syndrome". Integr Med Res 2019;8(2):89–91.
11. Stadje R, Dornieden K, Baum E, et al. The differential diagnosis of tiredness: a systematic review. BMC Fam Pract 2016;17(1).
12. Nijrolder I, Windt DAVD, Horst HEVD. Prognosis of Fatigue and Functioning in Primary Care: A 1-Year Follow-up Study. Ann Fam Med 2008;6(6):519–27.
13. Yurtsever C, Set T, Ateş E. The fatigue perception and its role in patient management. Dicle Tıp Dergisi 2018;77–84.
14. Zib M, Lim L, Walters W. Symptoms During Normal Pregnancy: A Prospective Controlled Study. Aust N Z J Obstet Gynaecol 1999;39(4):401–10.
15. Carlé A, Pedersen IB, Knudsen N, et al. Hypothyroid symptoms and the likelihood of overt thyroid failure: a population-based case–control study. Eur J Endocrinol 2014;171(5):593–602.
16. Canaris GJ, Steiner JF, Ridgway EC. Do traditional symptoms of hypothyroidism correlate with biochemical disease? J Gen Intern Med 1997;12(9):544–50.
17. Zulewski H. Estimation of Tissue Hypothyroidism by a New Clinical Score: Evaluation of Patients with Various Grades of Hypothyroidism and Controls. J Clin Endocrinol Metab 1997;82(3):771–6.
18. Nijrolder I, Windt DVD, Horst HVD. Prediction of outcome in patients presenting with fatigue in primary care. Br J Gen Pract 2009;59(561):101–9.
19. Chiu HY, Chen PY, Chuang LP, et al. Diagnostic accuracy of the Berlin questionnaire, STOP-BANG, STOP, and Epworth sleepiness scale in detecting obstructive sleep apnea: A bivariate meta-analysis. Sleep Med Rev 2017;36:57–70.

20. Chung F, Abdullah HR, Liao P. STOP-bang questionnaire a practical approach to screen for obstructive sleep apnea. Chest 2016;149(3):631–8.
21. Corfield EC, Martin NG, Nyholt DR. Co-occurrence and symptomatology of fatigue and depression. Compr Psychiatry 2016;71:1–10.
22. Levis B, Benedetti A, Thombs BD. Accuracy of Patient Health Questionnaire-9 (PHQ-9) for screening to detect major depression: Individual participant data meta-analysis. BMJ 2019;365:l1476.
23. Neuberger GB. Measures of fatigue: The Fatigue Questionnaire, Fatigue Severity Scale, Multidimensional Assessment of Fatigue Scale, and Short Form-36 Vitality (Energy/Fatigue) Subscale of the Short Form Health Survey. Arthritis Rheum 2003;49(S5):S175–83.
24. Rosenthal TC, Majeroni BA, Pretorius R, et al. Fatigue: An overview. Am Fam Physician 2008;78(10):1173–9.
25. Favrat B, Jacques C. Evaluation of fatigue. BMJ Best Pract 2020. Available at: https://bestpractice.bmj.com/topics/en-us/571.
26. Popp RFJ, Fierlbeck AK, Knüttel H, et al. Daytime sleepiness versus fatigue in patients with multiple sclerosis: A systematic review on the Epworth sleepiness scale as an assessment tool. Sleep Med Rev 2017;32:95–108.
27. Peterson TM, Peterson TW, Emerson S, et al. Coverage of CFS within U.S. medical schools. Universal Journal of Public Health 2013;1(4):177–9.
28. IOM (Institute of Medicine). Beyond myalgic encephalomyelitis/chronic fatigue syndrome: redefining an illness. Washington (DC): National Academies Press (US); 2015.
29. Jason L, Torres-Harding S, Njok M. CFIDS chronicle. In: The face of CFS in the U.S. 2006. p. 16–21.
30. CFIDS (Chronic Fatigue and Immune Dysfunction Syndrome) Association of America. ME/CFS road to diagnosis survey. Charlotte (NC): CFIDS Association of America; 2014.
31. Jason LA, Richman JA. How science can stigmatize: The case of chronic fatigue syndrome. J Chronic Fatigue Syndr 2008;14(4):85–103.
32. Carruthers BM, van de Sande MI. Myalgic encephalomyelitis/chronic fatigue syndrome: a clinical case definition and guidelines for medical practitioners: an overview of the Canadian consensus document. Vancouver (BC): Carruthers and van de Sande; 2005.
33. Corbitt M, Eaton-Fitch N, Staines D, et al. A systematic review of cytokines in chronic fatigue syndrome/myalgic encephalomyelitis/systemic exertion intolerance disease (CFS/ME/SEID). BMC Neurol 2019;19(1):207.
34. Chu L, Valencia IJ, Garvert DW, et al. Deconstructing post-exertional malaise in myalgic encephalomyelitis/chronic fatigue syndrome: A patient-centered, cross-sectional survey. PLoS One 2018;13:e0197811.
35. Sharpe M, Hawton K, Simkin S, et al. Cognitive behaviour therapy for the chronic fatigue syndrome: a randomized controlled trial. BMJ 1996;312:22.

Best Practices in the Management of Overweight and Obesity

Beverly G. Tchang, MD, Katherine H. Saunders, MD,
Leon I. Igel, MD*

KEYWORDS

- Weight • Overweight • Obesity • Antiobesity medication • Bariatric surgery • Diet
- Nutrition • Exercise

KEY POINTS

- Obesity is caused by dysregulated energy homeostasis pathways that encourage the accumulation of adiposity, which in turn results in the development or exacerbation of weight-related comorbidities.
- Obesity is a chronic disease that requires lifelong management.
- Weight reduction provides additional benefits for multiple comorbidities.
- Optimizing nutrition and physical activity is crucial to weight loss success.
- Pharmacotherapy or bariatric interventions can help patients achieve clinically significant weight loss when added to lifestyle modification.

INTRODUCTION

In 1998, the National Institutes of Health (NIH) recognized obesity as a disease, acknowledging its profound effects on individual health outcomes and socioeconomic costs.[1] The prevalence of obesity in the United States was 39.8% in 2015 to 2016[2] and is projected to be 48.9% by 2030.[3] It is linked to increased mortality and risks of cardiovascular disease (CVD), stroke, type 2 diabetes (T2D), and cancer.[4,5]

CAUSES AND PATHOPHYSIOLOGY

Obesity is caused by a state of neurohormonal imbalances in energy homeostasis that results in the development and defense of excess adiposity.[6] The hypothalamus is the

Disclosures: Dr B.G. Tchang has nothing to disclose. Dr K.H. Saunders reports personal fees from Intellihealth, outside the submitted work. Dr L.I. Igel reports personal fees from Novo Nordisk, outside the submitted work.
Department of Internal Medicine, Division of Endocrinology, Weill Cornell Medical College, 1165 York Avenue, New York, NY 10065, USA
* Corresponding author.
E-mail address: lei9004@med.cornell.edu

Med Clin N Am 105 (2021) 149–174
https://doi.org/10.1016/j.mcna.2020.08.018
0025-7125/21/© 2020 Elsevier Inc. All rights reserved.

medical.theclinics.com

primary center of energy regulation that communicates with the periphery to assess short-term and long-term energy status. It contains 2 populations of neurons that exert opposing effects on eating behavior (**Fig. 1**):

1. Orexigenic (increase appetite): agouti-related peptide (AgRP) and neuropeptide Y (NPY)
2. Anorexigenic (decrease appetite): proopiomelanocortin (POMC) and cocaine and amphetamine–regulated transcript (CART)

Rodent studies have shown that high-calorie diets cause inflammation in the hypothalamus and a reduction in POMC neurons.[7] In the periphery, adipocytes produce the anorexigenic hormone leptin to indicate the status of long-term energy reserves (ie, fat storage). Gastrointestinal (GI) peptides such as glucagonlike peptide-1 (GLP-1) signal the fed state by activating POMC/CART or suppressing AgRP/NPY. Ghrelin, the only known peripheral orexigenic hormone, stimulates AgRP.

The onset and severity of obesity caused by these pathophysiologic mechanisms are determined by genetics and the environment. The heritability of obesity, represented by body mass index (BMI), ranges from 40% to 70%.[6] Evolutions in food marketing and production, portion sizes, and occupation-related decreases in physical activity have also been identified as factors contributing to obesity.

Obesity is associated with several chronic diseases, with 2 predominant mechanisms to explain these effects: (1) mass effect and (2) adiposopathy.[8] In the former, the severity of diseases such as knee osteoarthritis and obesity hypoventilation syndrome are a direct response of the body to the weight of fat mass. In the latter,

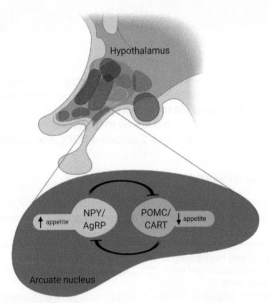

Fig. 1. Arcuate nucleus. The arcuate nucleus of the hypothalamus contains orexigenic (*yellow*) and anorexigenic (*red*) neurons that increase or decrease appetite. By communicating with the periphery, this nucleus is the primary energy homeostatic center of the brain. (*Courtesy of* Biorender, Toronto, Canada; with permission.) AgRP, Agouti-related peptide; CART, cocaine and amphetamine–regulated transcript; NPY, neuropeptide Y; POMC, proopiomelanocortin.

proinflammatory and prothrombotic cytokines, produced in the ischemic microenvironment of hypertrophic visceral adipocytes, lead to diseases such as T2D and CVD.

Clinical Evaluation

History
The clinical evaluation of a patient presenting for obesity management uses the standard interview process of the history of present illness (HPI), past medical history (PMH), past surgical history (PSH), social history, family history, medications, physical examination, and laboratory data.

The HPI should include a chronologic story of the patient's weight history that includes onset, duration, and precipitating and mitigating factors (**Table 1**). These open-ended questions allow the clinician to learn about the patient's behaviors while also providing an opportunity to explore the patient's nutrition knowledge, relationship with food, physical activity level, and life stressors.[9] PMH should focus on the identification of comorbidities associated with obesity, secondary causes of obesity, and potential contributors to obesity,[10] with the recognition that many of these relationships may be bidirectional[4] (**Box 1**).

PSH should include bariatric interventions (discussed later). Social history should include evaluation of nightshift work, pregnancy plans, smoking cessation, alcohol consumption, marijuana-induced hyperphagia, and stimulant use. Family history can assess the relative contribution of genetics versus environment to an individual's obesity and overall health status. Medication reconciliation must include both prescribed and over-the-counter medications because drug-induced weight gain is common and often missed (**Table 2**).[11]

Physical examination
Examination of patients with obesity includes standard blood pressure, heart rate, height, and weight measurements. Blood pressure cuffs of varied sizes and lengths should be available. Scales and examination room furniture with adequate weight capacities are also essential. Obesity severity is categorized by BMI class (**Table 3**), which may be adjusted for specific ethnic groups.[12] Because BMI does not distinguish between fat and muscle mass and does not account for distribution of adiposity, other measures of obesity that correlate to morbidity[5] have been entering clinical use, including waist circumference (WC), waist/hip ratio, and body fat percentage. WC is used to diagnose abdominal obesity, one of the components of the metabolic syndrome (see **Table 1**), and is commonly measured at the level of the anterior superior iliac spine.[1] The physical examination may require modification because standard techniques of inspection, palpation, and auscultation may be restricted by reduced mobility and increased subcutaneous adipose tissue. Practical suggestions for performing the examination include low-set examination tables, armless chairs, and enlisting the help of medical assistants for proper positioning. The clinician should look for signs of obesity-related complications (**Table 4**).

Laboratory data
Objective data to assess a patient's metabolic risk are a necessary component of the clinical evaluation (**Table 5**). Complete blood count and a comprehensive metabolic panel are essential. Patients should be screened for dyslipidemia and T2D.[4] Because thyroid-stimulating hormone (TSH) level is easily obtained and a higher prevalence of hypothyroidism exists in patients with obesity, TSH can be checked.[10] Assessment for other secondary causes of obesity and obesity-related comorbidities should be performed only if clinical suspicion exists.

Table 1
Initial evaluation of patients with obesity

HPI	General Questions
—	How did weight come to be a problem for you?
—	How long have you struggled with your weight?
—	Did any life events contribute to the weight issue? Onset after a diagnosis or initiation of a medication? Weights during or after high school, college, marriage, or pregnancy? Changes in employment or where you live? Weight gain around menopause?
—	What are the biggest challenges you face in losing weight or maintaining weight loss?
—	What has worked in the past to help you lose weight? Have you ever used medications for weight loss? Have you ever had weight loss surgery?
—	What is your lifetime weight range (nonpregnant)?
	Nutrition
—	Do you follow any special diet or have diet limitations for any reason?
—	How many meals per week do you eat in restaurants/order takeout?
—	What is your largest meal of the day?
—	Do you currently or have you ever had an eating disorder? Do you feel out of control when eating? Do you eat large volumes in a short period of time (binge)? Do you ever wake up in the middle of the night and eat?
	Physical Activity
—	What is your general activity level? How do you get to work?
—	Do you have an exercise routine?
—	Do you have any physical issues limiting your ability to be more active, other than weight?
PMH	**Secondary Causes or Contributors**
—	Single-gene mutations: leptin deficiency, MC4R deficiency Genetic syndromes: Prader-Willi Medications (see **Table 2**)
—	Cushing syndrome
—	Hypothyroidism
—	Male hypogonadism
—	Estrogen deficiency (menopause or premature ovarian failure)
—	PCOS
—	Growth hormone deficiency
	Physical Comorbidities
—	Metabolic syndrome

(continued on next page)

Table 1 (continued)	
HPI	**General Questions**

	• Waist circumference
	  ○ >102 cm (40″) (non-Asian male), >89 cm (35″) (non-Asian female)
	  ○ >89 cm (35″) (Asian male), >79 cm (31″) (Asian female)
	• Triglyceride levels ≥150 mg/dL or on triglyceride level–lowering medication
	• HDL level <40 mg/dL (male), <50 mg/dL (female), or on HDL level–increasing medication
	• Blood pressure ≥130/85 mm Hg or on antihypertensive agent
	• Fasting plasma glucose ≥100 mg/dL or on glucose level–lowering medication

—	Type 2 diabetes
—	Cardiovascular disease Hypertension Hyperlipidemia
—	Nonalcoholic fatty liver disease
—	Obstructive sleep apnea
—	Osteoarthritis
—	Cancer
	Psychological Comorbidities
—	Major depressive disorder
—	General anxiety disorder
—	Bipolar disorder, schizoaffective disorder, schizophrenia
—	Binge eating disorder
—	Anorexia nervosa, bulimia nervosa
PSH	Bariatric interventions Laparoscopic adjustable gastric band Laparoscopic sleeve gastrectomy Roux-en-Y gastric bypass Endoscopic sleeve gastroplasty Gastric balloon
Social history	Employment, shift work Sexual activity status, contraceptive use/method, and family planning Illicit substance use (eg, alcohol, smoking, marijuana, cocaine)
Family history	Obesity Type 2 diabetes, hyperlipidemia, hypertension, cardiovascular disease Cancer (especially medullary thyroid carcinoma)

Abbreviations: HDL, high-density lipoprotein; MC4R, melanocortin-4-receptor deficiency; PCOS, polycystic ovarian syndrome.
  Data from Refs.[4,10,62]

Management

Guidelines recommend the following goals for weight management:[4,5]

• BMI ≤ 30 kg/m² without comorbidities	Avoid weight gain
• BMI 25–29.9 kg/m² with comorbidities	5%–10% weight loss over 6 mo
• BMI ≥ 30 kg/m²	5%–10% weight loss over 6 mo

Box 1
Congestive heart failure and the obesity paradox

Some epidemiologic studies have suggested the existence of a so-called obesity paradox, in which higher BMIs are correlated to better outcomes in specific diseases, particularly congestive heart failure (CHF). Although experts unanimously agree that obesity increases the risk of incident CHF, once CHF is diagnosed mortalities seem to be lowest in the overweight and class I obesity ranges. However, subsequent investigations found that higher weights correlated with greater lean mass and better cardiorespiratory fitness, lending a potential explanation for the observed obesity paradox.

Data from Carbone S, Canada JM, Billingsley HE, Siddiqui MS, Elagizi A, Lavie CJ. Obesity paradox in cardiovascular disease: where do we stand? Vasc Health Risk Manag. 2019;15:89-100.

Depending on results from the diagnostic work-up, the clinician may be required to address secondary causes such as drug-induced weight gain (see **Table 2**) or refer to a specialist for endocrinologic disorders[10] and treatable genetic conditions.

Lifestyle modification

The foundation of obesity management is lifestyle modification. Intensive lifestyle interventions (ILIs) are classically structured as 14 sessions over 6 months that provide patients with education in nutrition, exercise, and behavior change.[5] The frequency of contact directly correlates to the magnitude of weight loss and durability of weight loss maintenance.

Nutrition

A caloric deficit is required for weight loss. Guidelines have recommended a daily caloric deficit of about 500 kcal,[4,5] which typically amounts to 1200 to 1500 kcal/d for women and 1500 to 1800 kcal/d for men. Very-low-calorie diets, defined as a caloric intake of 500 to 800 kcal/d, often use meal replacement shakes or bars and are effective short-term options that should be performed only under medical supervision.[5] More recently, a third strategy to achieve a hypocaloric diet has emerged, called intermittent fasting (IF). IF encompasses a variety of modalities in which individuals restrict their caloric intake based on time (eg, day of the week or time of day) (**Table 6**). Alternate-day fasting, in which "fasting" days of 500 to 800 kcal intake are alternated with usual intake, is comparable with continuous caloric restriction over 1 year.[13] Another option, called time-restricted feeding, reduces caloric intake by an average of 300 kcal/d when the window of consumption is condensed from 12 hours to 8 hours.[14]

The macronutrient composition of the ideal weight loss diet has been debated for decades. Robust data from randomized controlled trials (RCTs) of long duration[15,16] support the weight and health benefits of a low-fat diet, defined as less than or equal to 20% to 30% of total daily calories (**Table 7**).[5] For example, the Look Action for Health in Diabetes (Look AHEAD) trial showed that 50.3% of individuals randomized to ILI lost greater than or equal to 5% of baseline weight at 8 years, compared with 35.7% in the control group.[16] However, emerging evidence suggests that low-carbohydrate diets ($\leq$150 g/d) may have a metabolic advantage over low-fat diets because of reduction in insulin secretion[17] because insulin is anabolic and stimulates lipogenesis while suppressing lipolysis. Meta-analyses comparing low-carbohydrate with low-fat diets differ in their conclusions depending on the protocols of RCTs included.[18,19] Proponents of low-carbohydrate diets argue that their superiority is best demonstrated by the ketogenic diet, which establishes a nutritional ketosis via

Table 2
Drugs associated with weight gain and suggested alternatives

Category	Drug Class	Weight Gain	Alternatives
Psychiatry	Antipsychotics	Clozapine	Ziprasidone
		Risperidone	Lurasidone
		Olanzapine	
		Quetiapine	
		Haloperidol	
		Perphenazine	
		Quetiapine	
	Antidepressants/anxiolytics	TCAs	Bupropion[a]
		Amitriptyline	Fluoxetine
		Doxepin	Sertraline
		Imipramine	
		Nortriptyline	
		Trimipramine	
		Mirtazapine	
		SSRIs	
		Fluoxetine[b]	
		Sertraline[b]	
		Paroxetine	
		Fluvoxamine	
		MAOi	
		Phenelzine	
		Tranylcypromine	
	Mood stabilizer	Lithium	Topiramate[a]
Neurology	Anticonvulsants	Carbamazepine	Lamotrigine[b]
		Gabapentin	Topiramate[a]
		Valproate	Zonisamide
—	Sleep aids	Diphenhydramine-containing OTC agents	Melatonin
		Mirtazapine	Benzodiazepines
		Trazodone[b]	

(continued on next page)

Table 2
(continued)

Category	Drug Class	Weight Gain	Alternatives
Endocrinology	Diabetes medications	Insulin Sulfonylureas Thiazolidinediones Sitagliptin[b] Meglitinides	Metformin[a] Acarbose Miglitol Pramlintide[a] Exenatide[a] Dulaglutide[a] Liraglutide[a] Semaglutide[a] Canagliflozin[a] Dapagliflozin[a] Empagliflozin[a] Ertugliflozin[a]
Obstetrics and gynecology	Contraceptives	Progestational steroids Medroxyprogesterone Injection Etonogestrel implant Levonorgestrel IUD	Barrier methods Nonhormonal IUD
Cardiology	Antihypertensives	α-Blockers[b] β-Blockers[b]	Carvedilol[b] ACEis[b] CCBs[b] ARBs

Allergy and immunology	Antihistamines	Diphenhydramine Cetirizine[b] Levocetirizine[b] Fexofenadine[b] Doxepin[b] Cyproheptadine[b]	Loratadine Decongestants
	Immunosuppressants	Corticosteroids	NSAIDs Steroid inhalers[b]
Infectious disease	Antiretroviral therapy	Protease inhibitors	None

Abbreviations: ACEi, angiotensin-converting enzyme inhibitor; ARB, angiotensin-2 receptor blocker; CCBs, calcium channel blockers; IUD, intrauterine device; MAOi, monoamine oxidase inhibitor; NSAIDs, nonsteroidal antiinflammatory drugs; OTC, over the counter; SSRI, selective serotonin reuptake inhibitor; TCA, tricyclic antidepressants.

[a] Medications known to reduce weight.

[b] Medications with poor-quality or mixed evidence for weight gain.

Adapted from Apovian CM, Aronne LJ, Bessesen DH, et al. Pharmacological Management of Obesity: An Endocrine Society Clinical Practice Guideline. The Journal of clinical endocrinology and metabolism. 2015;100(2):342-362; with permission.

Table 3
Classes of body mass index

	BMI (kg/m^2)
Overweight	25.0–29.9
Obesity, class I	30.0–34.9
Obesity, class II	35.0–39.9
Obesity, class III	≥40.0

Data from National Heart Lung and Blood Institute. Clinical Guidelines on the Identification, Evaluation, and Treatment of Overweight and Obesity in Adults: The Evidence Report. Obesity Education Initiative. 1998;98-4083 and Garvey WT, Mechanick JI, Brett EM, et al. AMERICAN ASSOCIATION OF CLINICAL ENDOCRINOLOGISTS AND AMERICAN COLLEGE OF ENDOCRINOLOGY COMPREHENSIVE CLINICAL PRACTICE GUIDELINES FOR MEDICAL CARE OF PATIENTS WITH OBESITY. Endocrine practice: official journal of the American College of Endocrinology and the American Association of Clinical Endocrinologists. 2016;22 Suppl 3:1-203.

Table 4
Potential physical examination findings in patients with obesity

Domain	Possible Findings	Associated Comorbidity
Head and neck	Supracervical or supraclavicular fullness	Hypercortisolism
	Moon facies	Hypercortisolism
	Poor visualization of soft palate or uvula	OSA
Cardiovascular	Tachycardia or irregular heart beat	Atrial fibrillation
	Valvular murmur	CHF
Lung	Wheezing	Reactive airway disease
Abdomen	Hepatomegaly	NAFLD
	Predominant truncal adiposity	Insulin resistance
Gonadal	Vaginal atrophy	Menopause
	Small testicular size	Hypogonadism
Neurologic	Reduced distal sensation to light touch, temperature, or vibration	T2D
Musculoskeletal	Enlarged joints	OA
	Reduced range of motion	OA
	Proximal muscle weakness	Hypercortisolism
Skin and hair	Erythematous rash within skin folds	Cutaneous candidiasis
	Skin tags	Insulin resistance
	Velvety hyperpigmentation in skin folds	Acanthosis nigricans
	Hirsutism	PCOS
	Excess acne	PCOS
	Wide hyperpigmented striae	Hypercortisolism
	Edema	CHF

Abbreviations: CHF, congestive heart failure; NAFLD, nonalcoholic fatty liver disease; OA, osteoarthritis; OSA, obstructive sleep apnea.

Table 5
Laboratory screening evaluation in obesity

Recommended	Reason for Screening
CBC	Standard of care Platelet count is used in calculated risk scores for hepatic fibrosis
CMP	Standard of care Increased liver function tests may be the first sign of NAFLD

Lipid profile	Dyslipidemia, hyperlipidemia,
	   and hypertriglyceridemia are components
	   of the metabolic syndrome and have
	   high correlation with obesity/overweight
	Screening recommendations:
	USPSTF: age $\geq$ 20 y with obesity
	NCEP ATP III: age $\geq$ 20 y

Hemoglobin A1c	Prediabetes and T2D are components of
	   the metabolic syndrome and have
	   high correlation with obesity/overweight
	Screening recommendations:
	USPSTF: age $\geq$ 40 y with overweight or obesity
	ADA: overweight or obesity and
	   at least 1 additional risk factor

TSH	Low-cost test for potential secondary cause or contributor to weight gain
Not Recommended	**Reason for not Screening**

Total testosterone	High prevalence of false-positive caused
	   by low sex hormone binding globulin
	   level in obesity

Free testosterone	Low free testosterone level commonly improves
	   with weight loss and is not evidence
	   of an independent disease

Estradiol, luteinizing hormone,
   follicle-stimulating hormone
	Perimenopause and menopause have not been
	   definitively established as causative factors

Insulin	Both fasting and postprandial insulin levels
	   are highly dependent on
	   macronutrient composition
	   of recent dietary intake

Cortisol	Diurnal variations, circadian rhythm disruptions,
	   and environmental stressors cause
	   physiologic changes to cortisol levels and
	   do not necessarily represent
	   meaningful disorder

Leptin	Congenital leptin deficiency is an extremely rare monogenic obesity disorder

Abbreviations: ADA, American Diabetes Association; CBC, complete blood count; CMP, comprehensive metabolic panel; NCEP ATP III, National Cholesterol Education Program Adult Treatment Panel III; TSH, thyroid-stimulating hormone; USPSTF, United States Preventive Services Task Force.
Data from Refs.[63–66]

Table 6
Types of intermittent fasting

	Pattern of Eating
Alternate-day fast	Alternating days of hypocaloric intake with normal caloric intake
5:2	2 d/wk of hypocaloric intake (500–800 kcal/d), which can be consecutive or nonconsecutive
Fast mimicking	Hypocaloric intake (classically 600 kcal/d) for 5–14 d at a time, repeated monthly or as needed
Time-restricting feeding	Limiting daily caloric intake to designated hours of the day; caloric intake is not specified

Data from Refs.[13,14,67,68]

Table 7
Characteristics of common diets

	Carbohydrate	Fat	Protein
Macronutrient Restricted			
Low carbohydrate	≤150 g/d	Not standardized	Not standardized
Atkins	<20 g/d for 2 wk; can +5 g/d weekly for maintenance	Not standardized	High
Ketogenic	<20–50 g/d	High	Not standardized
Low fat	Not standardized	<20%–30%	Not standardized
Ornish	Not standardized	<10%	Not standardized
Diabetes Prevention Program	Not standardized	<30%	Not standardized
Zone	40%	30%	30%
Non–macronutrient Restricted			
DASH	Vegetables, fruits, whole grains, fat-free or low-fat dairy products, fish, poultry, beans, nuts, and vegetable oils		
Paleo	Vegetables, fruits, grass-produced meat, fish/seafood, eggs, nuts and seeds, nut/seed/fruit oils		
Vegan	No meat or animal products		
Vegetarian	No meat. Secondary animal products such as eggs, dairy, and cheese are allowed		
Pescatarian	Vegetarian with the allowance for fish		
Flexitarian	Mostly plant-based foods with occasional meat and animal products		

Abbreviation: DASH, Dietary Approaches to Stop Hypertension.
Data from U.S. News & World Report, Best Diets 2020. Available at: https://health.usnews.com/best-diet. Accessed on February 25, 2020.

high fat and very low carbohydrate consumption,[20] but long-term studies show poor adherence.[21] Diets that avoid specific macronutrient restriction, such as the Mediterranean diet[22] and MyPlate,[23] also have health benefits. Given the variety of dietary options, researchers have found weight loss efficacy is best predicted by adherence, not macronutrient composition.[24]

General consensus on the optimal timing of food intake seems to be that earlier is better.[25] A larger breakfast instead of a larger dinner results in more weight loss,[26] and earlier lunches or dinners result in better insulin-glucose profiles.[27,28] However, the addition of breakfast in individuals already skipping breakfast does not reduce evening caloric intake and may cause weight gain.[29]

Physical activity

The role of physical activity in weight management is 2-fold: to support an energy deficit and to preserve lean muscle mass. Total energy expenditure (TEE) is partitioned into basal metabolic rate (BMR), diet-induced thermogenesis (DIT), nonexercise activity thermogenesis (NEAT), and exercise (**Fig. 2**). Exercise, both cardiovascular and resistance training (RT), is the only component of TEE that is significantly modifiable. The combination of diet and exercise always results in greater weight loss than either modality alone.

The American College of Sports Medicine (ACSM) provides evidence-based recommendations for cardiovascular exercise to prevent weight gain, achieve weight loss, and maintain weight loss:[30]

• Weight maintenance	150–250 min/wk
• Weight loss	>150–420 min/wk
• Weight loss maintenance	200–300 min/wk

The individual's response to exercise is dose responsive and heterogeneous. For example, the landmark Midwest Exercise Trial-1 showed that a prescription of 225 min/wk of moderate-intensity cardiovascular exercise allowed most men to lose weight, but roughly 50% of women gained weight.[31]

RT plays an important role in weight loss maintenance because it preserves lean muscle mass, which determines BMR, and weight loss is accompanied by a reduction in BMR.[32] RT mitigates lean muscle loss in weight loss[30] and increases BMR and lean muscle mass when applied without a hypocaloric diet.[33,34]

Behavior

In addition to nutrition and physical activity modifications, behavioral changes also assist in weight loss success. Behavioral interventions are often delivered on a scheduled basis (eg, weekly or monthly education sessions) in person or electronically,[35] and can be in an individual or group setting. The tenets of behavioral treatment of obesity are goal setting, self-monitoring, and stimulus control (**Table 8**),[36] which have been shown to be beneficial in weight loss and weight loss maintenance.[37,38]

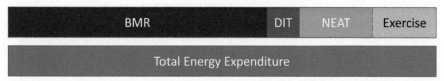

Fig. 2. Components of TEE. BMR is the largest contributor to TEE and cannot be directly modulated by daily activities. The types of physical activity, NEAT and exercise, are targets of many interventions to increase TEE.

Table 8		
Behavioral treatment of obesity		
Goal Setting	**Self-monitoring**	**Stimulus Control**
• Goals should be specific and feasible	• Food logging increases awareness of caloric and macronutrient intake	• Patients learn to modify external cues to create an environment more conducive to behavior change
• Individuals should report their successes or challenges at every session	• Electronic activity monitoring devices provide information about energy expenditure	• Uses problem-solving strategies, cognitive restructuring, stress management
• Promotes accountability	• Frequent weighing is associated with better weight loss maintenance	• Stress-related eating behaviors (binge eating, comfort eating, emotional eating) may require collaboration with psychologist or psychiatrist

Data from Butryn ML, Webb V, Wadden TA. Behavioral treatment of obesity. Psychiatr Clin North Am. 2011;34(4):841-859 and Burke LE, Wang J, Sevick MA. Self-Monitoring in Weight Loss: A Systematic Review of the Literature. J Am Diet Assoc. 2011;111(1):92-102.

Pharmacotherapy

Pharmacotherapy for weight loss (**Table 9**) should be considered to help patients achieve targeted weight loss and health goals as an adjunct to comprehensive lifestyle intervention for individuals who are motivated to lose weight and have a BMI greater than or equal to 30 kg/m^2 or a BMI greater than or equal to 27 kg/m^2 with at least 1 obesity-associated comorbidity (eg, T2D, hypertension, hyperlipidemia, and obstructive sleep apnea).[39] The rationale for adding antiobesity medication (AOM) to lifestyle modifications is 2-fold:

1. To help patients adhere to a lower-calorie diet more consistently to achieve weight loss and improve health[5]
2. To directly address the pathophysiologic mechanisms that cause weight gain and the metabolic adaptations that drive weight regain[32,40]

Before starting a medication for weight loss, it is important to discuss with patients that obesity is a chronic disease that may require long-term treatment.

Phentermine

Phentermine is an adrenergic agonist that leads to weight loss by activation of the sympathetic nervous system with a subsequent decrease in appetite and increase in BMR.[41,42] It remains the most frequently prescribed AOM. Phentermine as a monotherapy is only US Food and Drug Administration (FDA)–approved for short-term use (3 months), but, in clinical practice, many practitioners prescribe it for a longer duration. The recommended dosage of phentermine is 15 to 37.5 mg orally once daily in the morning.[43] Low-dose phentermine is available as a scored 8-mg tablet that can be prescribed up to 3 times per day.

Optimal candidates for phentermine include patients with obesity who need assistance with appetite suppression. Because of the mild increase in heart rate and/or

Table 9
Summary of antiobesity medications

Medication (Year Approved)	Mechanism of Action and Typical Dosage	Trial	Trial Arms	Average Weight Loss (%)	≥5% TBW (%)	≥10% TBW (%)	Most Common Side Effects
Phentermine (1959, schedule IV controlled substance)	Adrenergic agonist Typical dosing: 8–37.5 mg QAM	Aronne et al[43] 28 wk	15 mg daily	6.1[a]	46.2	20.8	Dry mouth, difficulty sleeping, irritability
			7.5 mg daily	5.5[a]	43.3	12.5	
			Placebo	1.7	15.5	6.8	
			[a]Topiramate ER and phentermine/ topiramate ER arms excluded				
Orlistat (1999)	Lipase inhibitor Typical dosing: 60–120 mg TID with meals	XENDOS 208 wk	120 mg TID (week 52)	9.6[a]	72.8	41.0	Fecal urgency, oily stool, flatus with discharge, fecal incontinence
			120 mg TID (week 208)	5.3[a]	52.8	26.2	
			Placebo (week 52)	5.6	45.1	20.8	
			Placebo (week 208)	2.7	37.3	15.6	
Phentermine/ topiramate ER (2012, schedule IV controlled substance)	Adrenergic agonist/ neurostabilizer Typical dose titration: 3.75/23 mg daily for 2 wk, increasing to 7.5/46 mg daily, with further dose escalation as needed/ tolerated thereafter	EQUIP 56 wk	15/92 mg daily	10.9[a]	66.7	47.2	Paresthesia, dizziness, dysgeusia, insomnia, constipation, dry mouth
			3.75/23 mg daily	5.1[a]	44.9	18.8	
			Placebo	1.6	17.3	7.4	
		CONQUER 56 wk	15/92 mg daily	9.8[a]	70.0	47.6	
			7.5/46 mg daily	7.8[a]	62.1	37.3	
			Placebo	1.2	20.8	7.4	
		SEQUEL 108 wk (52-wk extension of CONQUER trial)	15/92 mg daily	10.5[a]	79.3	53.9	
			7.5/46 mg daily	9.3[a]	75.2	50.3	
			Placebo	1.8	30.0	11.5	

(continued on next page)

Table 9
(continued)

Medication (Year Approved)	Mechanism of Action and Typical Dosage	Trial	Trial Arms	Average Weight Loss (%) Data from weeks 0–108	≥5% TBW (%)	≥10% TBW (%)	Most Common Side Effects
Naltrexone/bupropion ER (2014)	Opioid receptor antagonist/dopamine and norepinephrine reuptake inhibitor Typical dose titration: Week 1: 8/90 mg QAM Week 2: 8/90 mg BID Week 3:16/180 mg QAM, 8/90 mg QPM Week 4 (and beyond): 16/180 mg BID	COR-I 56 wk	16/180 mg BID	6.1[a]	48.0	24.6	Nausea, constipation, headache, dizziness, insomnia, dry mouth
			8/180 mg BID	5.0[a]	39.5	20.2	
			Placebo	1.3	16.4	7.4	
		COR-II 56 wk	16/180 mg BID	6.4[a]	50.2	28.3	
			Placebo	1.2	17.1	5.7	
		COR-BMOD 56 wk	16/180 mg BID	9.3[a]	66.4	41.5	
			Placebo	5.1	42.5	20.2	
		COR-DIABETES 56 wk	16/180 mg BID	5.0[a]	44.5	18.5	
			Placebo	1.8	18.9	5.7	
Liraglutide 3.0 mg (2014)	GLP-1 receptor agonist Typical dose titration: Week 1: 0.6 mg daily Week 2: 1.2 mg daily Week 3: 1.8 mg daily Week 4: 2.4 mg daily Week 5 (and beyond): 3.0 mg daily	SCALE Obesity and Prediabetes 56 wk	3.0 mg daily	8.0[a]	63.2	33.1	Nausea, vomiting, diarrhea, constipation, dyspepsia, abdominal pain
			Placebo	2.6	27.1	10.6	
		SCALE Diabetes 56 wk	3.0 mg daily	6[a]	54.3	25.2	
			1.8 mg daily	4.7[a]	40.4	15.9	
			Placebo	2.0	21.4	6.7	
		SCALE Maintenance 56 wk (after initial ≥5% weight loss with LCD)	3.0 mg daily	6.2[a]	50.5	26.1	
			Placebo	0.2	21.8	6.3	

Abbreviations: BID, twice daily; ER, extended release; LCD, low-calorie diet; QAM, every morning; QPM, every evening; TBW, total body weight; TID, thrice daily; XENDOS, Xenical in the Prevention of Diabetes in Obese Subjects.

[a] *P*<.001 versus placebo.

Adapted from Igel LI, Kumar RB, Saunders KH, Aronne LJ. Practical Use of Pharmacotherapy for Obesity. Gastroenterology. 2017 Feb 9. pii: S0016-5085(17)30142-7; with permission.

blood pressure that can accompany phentermine use, this medication is generally used in younger patients without evidence of unstable coronary disease or uncontrolled hypertension. Patients who have anxiety or insomnia may find these conditions exacerbated by phentermine and would not be ideal candidates.

Orlistat

Orlistat promotes weight loss by inhibiting gastrointestinal lipases, thereby decreasing the absorption of fat from the gastrointestinal tract. Orlistat 120 mg ingested 3 times per day with meals decreases fat absorption by approximately 30%.[44] Half-strength orlistat (60 mg) ingested 3 times daily is approved for over-the-counter use.

Orlistat can lead to gastrointestinal side effects, which can often be ameliorated by following a balanced, reduced-calorie diet with no more than ~30% of calories from fat at any meal.[45] The addition of a fiber supplement can also be helpful. Orlistat decreases the absorption of fat-soluble vitamins (A, D, E, and K), and patients should be instructed to take a multivitamin (separately from the medication) to ensure adequate nutrition.

Optimal candidates for orlistat use include patients with obesity and constipation and/or concomitant hypercholesterolemia. Orlistat is contraindicated in patients with malabsorptive syndromes or cholestasis.

Phentermine/topiramate extended release

Phentermine/topiramate extended release (ER) combines the sympathomimetic amine phentermine (discussed earlier) with topiramate ER. Topiramate monotherapy is FDA approved for epilepsy as well as migraine prophylaxis and has been found to decrease caloric intake and reduce cravings via GABA (gamma-aminobutyric acid) and glutamate modulation as well as carbonic anhydrase inhibition. The combination of phentermine plus topiramate ER leads to additive weight loss by targeting different appetite pathways simultaneously. Phentermine/topiramate is available in 4 doses: 3.75/23 mg, 7.5/46 mg, 11.25/69 mg, and 15/92 mg.

Ideal candidates for phentermine/topiramate ER include younger patients with obesity (because older patients may have undiagnosed heart disease that could potentially be worsened by sympathomimetics) and patients with concomitant migraines who could benefit from the appetite suppressant effects of the agent. Because of the phentermine component, this medication should not be prescribed to patients with a history of CVD or other conditions that could be exacerbated by a stimulant. In addition, because of teratogenicity associated with topiramate, the FDA requires a risk evaluation and mitigation strategy to inform prescribers and female patients of reproductive potential about the possible increased risk of orofacial clefts in infants exposed to topiramate during the first trimester of pregnancy.[46–48]

Naltrexone/bupropion extended release

Naltrexone/bupropion combines the dopamine/norepinephrine reuptake inhibitor bupropion with the opioid antagonist naltrexone. Bupropion monotherapy is FDA approved as an antidepressant and to assist with smoking cessation. Inhibiting reuptake of dopamine and norepinephrine modulates the central reward pathways triggered by food. Naltrexone monotherapy is FDA approved for the treatment of alcohol and opioid dependence. Naltrexone antagonizes an inhibitory feedback loop that would otherwise limit bupropion's anorectic properties, and the combination of naltrexone/bupropion has been shown to activate POMC neurons in the arcuate nucleus of the hypothalamus.[49]

Naltrexone/bupropion should be avoided in patients with uncontrolled hypertension, uncontrolled pain, history of seizures, or any condition that predisposes to seizure, such as anorexia or bulimia nervosa, or abrupt discontinuation of alcohol, benzodiazepines, barbiturates, or antiepileptic drugs. Bupropion carries a black box warning related to a potential increase in suicidal thoughts in young adults (< 24 years old) within the first few months of treatment initiation, and patients should be monitored closely for any mood changes (although no evidence of suicidality was reported in phase III studies).[50–53]

Ideal candidates for naltrexone/bupropion include patients who describe strong cravings for food and/or addictive behaviors related to food. Patients who have concomitant depression, are trying to quit smoking or decrease alcohol consumption are also good candidates.

Liraglutide 3.0

Liraglutide is a GLP-1 receptor agonist that is also FDA approved for the treatment of T2D in doses up to 1.8 mg daily. Liraglutide works both centrally (eg, the hypothalamus) and in the gastrointestinal tract to delay gastric emptying and decrease food intake as well as subjective hunger.[54,55]

Liraglutide carries a black box warning related to an association with medullary thyroid cancer (MTC) in rodents, although the relevance to humans has not been determined. Nonetheless, liraglutide is contraindicated in patients who have had MTC or who have a family history of multiple endocrine neoplasia type 2.[55] Concomitant use of liraglutide with insulin or insulin secretagogues increases the risk of hypoglycemia.

Ideal patients for liraglutide include those with overweight or obesity who report inadequate meal satiety, and/or have T2D, prediabetes, or impaired glucose tolerance. Liraglutide is not appropriate for patients with an aversion to needles, because it requires a daily subcutaneous injection.

Bariatric surgery and devices

Bariatric surgery results in greater improvement in weight loss outcomes and weight-associated comorbidities compared with nonsurgical interventions.[56] The 3 most commonly performed procedures in the United States are the laparoscopic sleeve gastrectomy (LSG), the Roux-en-Y gastric bypass (RYGB), and the laparoscopic adjustable gastric band (LAGB) (**Table 10**).[57] Bariatric surgery should be considered in patients who are motivated to lose weight but have not achieved sufficient weight loss for target health goals following behavioral treatment, with or without pharmacotherapy.[57] Patients should have a BMI greater than or equal to 40 kg/m^2 or a BMI greater than or equal to 35 kg/m^2 with at least 1 significant obesity-related comorbid condition, such as obstructive sleep apnea.[58]

The LSG and RYGB are performed more frequently than the LAGB because they are associated with greater weight reduction, better management of obesity-associated comorbidities, and fewer adverse events.[5] Contraindications include poor adherence to medical treatment, severe psychological disorders, and illnesses that significantly reduce life expectancy and are unlikely to improve with weight loss. Better outcomes are achieved when patients commit to long-term lifestyle changes and medical follow-up; however, most patients regain some weight.

Laparoscopic sleeve gastrectomy

LSG removes ~70% of the stomach along the greater curvature. The fundus, which secretes the hunger hormone ghrelin, is removed. The remaining stomach is shaped like a sleeve and the pyloric sphincter remains intact. There is a lower risk of nutritional deficiencies with LSG compared with RYGB, and LSG is associated with fewer

Table 10
Most commonly performed bariatric surgeries

Procedure	Description	Total Body Weight Loss at One Year (%)	Reversibility	Procedures Performed in 2018 (%)
LSG	~70% of stomach removed along greater curvature	25	No	61.4
RYGB	Small pouch (~<50 mL) created from proximal stomach and attached to jejunum, bypasses most of stomach, duodenum, and most of jejunum	30	Yes (rarely done)	17.0
LAGB	Inflatable silicone band placed around fundus of stomach to create small pouch (~30 mL); pouch capacity adjusted by increasing or decreasing quantity of saline in band via subcutaneous port	15–20	Yes	1.1

Data from Heymsfield SB, Wadden TA. Mechanisms, pathophysiology, and management of obesity. N Engl J Med. 2017;376:254-266 and American Society for Metabolic and Bariatric Surgery. Estimate of Bariatric Surgery Numbers, 2011-2018. Available at: https://asmbs.org/resources/estimate-of-bariatric-surgery-numbers. Accessed February 24, 2020.

complications than RYGB and LAGB. Early adverse events include bleeding, stenosis, leakage at the staple line, reflux, and vomiting; late complications include stomach expansion, which can lead to decreased restriction.[56] Unlike RYGB and LAGB, LSG is not reversible.

Roux-en-Y gastric bypass
In the RYGB, a small pouch is created from the proximal stomach and attached to the jejunum, thereby bypassing the rest of the stomach, the duodenum, and most of the jejunum. There is a lower rate of gastroesophageal reflux following RYGB compared with LSG; RYGB can often improve symptoms of reflux. Early adverse events include obstruction, stricture, leakage, and failure of the staple line; late adverse events include anastomosis ulceration and nutritional deficiencies.[56] Dumping syndrome can develop at any time. The RYGB is technically reversible; however, it is generally only reversed in extreme situations.

Laparoscopic adjustable gastric band
The LAGB is an inflatable band that is placed around the fundus of the stomach in order to produce a small, proximal pouch. The capacity of the pouch is adjusted by adding or removing saline to the band through a subcutaneous port. Although the procedure is reversible and less invasive than LSG and RYGB, many bands are eventually removed because of insufficient weight loss and/or complications.[59] The most common adverse events include nausea, vomiting, reflux, obstruction, band erosion, and band migration.[60]

Antiobesity devices

Devices are emerging as options for the treatment of obesity (**Table 11**). Not only are they minimally invasive and reversible but they are potentially more effective than AOMs, generally safer for poor surgical candidates, and possibly less expensive than bariatric surgery.[61] The 5 FDA-approved devices are 2 intragastric balloons, an aspiration device, superabsorbent hydrogel capsules, and the TransPyloric Shuttle. Although the devices are not widely used currently, they may become more widespread in the future as more health care providers are trained to use them and insurance coverage improves.

Table 11				
Devices approved for overweight and obesity by the Food and Drug Administration				
Device (Year Approved)	**BMI Indication (kg/m²)**	**Description**	**Total Body Weight Loss (%)**	**Duration of Intervention (mo)**
Orbera Intragastric Balloon (2015)	30–40	Endoscopically placed intragastric balloon filled with 400–700 mL of saline, removed endoscopically after 6 mo	Device: 10.2 Sham: 3.3	6
Obalon Balloon System (2016)	30–40	3 sequentially swallowed balloons filled with 250 mL of gas each, removed endoscopically 6 mo after first balloon placed	Device: 6.6 Sham: 3.4	6
AspireAssist (2016)	35–55	Endoscopically placed percutaneous gastrostomy aspiration tube; 30% of each meal removed from the stomach	Device: 12.1 Lifestyle alone[a]:3.5	12
Plenity (2019)	25–40	Capsules containing superabsorbent hydrogel, occupy one-quarter of stomach volume when hydrated, 3 capsules (2.25 g/dose) administered with water before lunch and dinner	Device: 6.4 Placebo: 4.4	6
TransPyloric Shuttle (2019)	30–40	Endoscopically placed device comprising a large spherical bulb (above pylorus) attached to small cylindrical weight (moves freely in duodenum); removed endoscopically after 12 mo	Device: 9.5 Sham: 2.8	12

[a] Lifestyle comprises diet and exercise counseling.
Data from Refs.[69–80]

Intragastric balloons

Intragastric balloons are space-occupying devices that are placed in the stomach to reduce functional gastric volume. The Orbera balloon is placed endoscopically and filled with 400 to 700 mL of saline. After 6 months, it is removed endoscopically. The Obalon balloon system comprises 3 balloons, which are swallowed as capsules sequentially over 3 months. Each balloon is filled with 250 mL of gas. Six months after the first balloon is placed, the 3 balloons are removed endoscopically.

Aspiration therapy

The AspireAssist device consists of a percutaneous gastrostomy tube that is placed endoscopically and attached to an external aspiration port positioned at the abdominal surface. Patients must chew thoroughly and drink sufficient liquid with each meal so that food particles are 5 mm or less in diameter to flow through the gastrostomy tube in a slurry. After each meal, patients aspirate 30% of ingested food.

Hydrogel capsules

Plenity is a capsule composed of superabsorbent hydrogel particles. When capsules are taken with water before a meal, they can absorb up to 100 times their weight in water to occupy a quarter of average stomach volume. The recommended dose is 3 capsules (2.25 g/dose) before lunch and dinner.

TransPyloric Shuttle

The TransPyloric Shuttle is a device composed of a large spherical bulb connected to a small cylindrical weight. Following endoscopic placement, an overtube facilitates coiling of a silicone cord into the bulb. Although the weight moves freely in the duodenum, the bulb remains above the pylorus to prevent migration. Peristaltic contractions result in intermittent gastric outlet obstruction and delayed gastric emptying.

Future directions

Although the primary tools of obesity management remain lifestyle modification, pharmacotherapy, and bariatric interventions, the future of obesity medicine is rapidly evolving to accommodate the variety of patients who present for weight management. Nutrition science is investigating genome-based diets to provide precision medicine and is finding nutrient sequencing (ie, the order in which macronutrients are ingested) can also affect hormonal responses and weight management. The microbiome is playing a growing role in how energy regulation is understood. AOMs are expanding to include triple agonists/antagonists to address the multiple pathophysiologic mechanisms that drive weight gain. New nonsurgical bariatric interventions, such as the endoscopic sleeve gastroplasty, are also emerging tools. The future of obesity management is progressing toward multimodal approaches that optimize the complimentary effects of lifestyle changes, medications, and procedures.

SUMMARY

Obesity is a chronic disease caused by dysregulated energy homeostasis pathways that encourage the accumulation of adiposity, which, in turn, results in the development or exacerbation of weight-related comorbidities. Treatment of obesity relies on a foundation of lifestyle modification. Weight loss pharmacotherapy, bariatric surgeries, and novel devices are additional tools to help patients achieve their health and weight goals. Appropriate management of patients with obesity provides multiple metabolic benefits beyond weight loss.

CLINICS CARE POINTS

- Obesity is a chronic disease caused by dysfunctional communication pathways between hypothalamic and peripheral orexigenic and anorexigenic signals, which is propagated by both genetics and environmental stressors.
- Treatment of obesity requires lifelong management, but the metabolic benefits of weight reduction extend beyond weight loss alone.
- Because many diets have been shown to be effective for weight loss, nutrition advice should be individualized to each patient to optimize adherence.
- Aerobic exercise and RT are tools to support weight loss, weight maintenance, and general health.
- AOMs help patients achieve clinically significant weight loss when added to lifestyle modification; the choice of AOM depends on the potential benefits and side effects in each individual.
- Bariatric surgery is an option for eligible patients with proven efficacy and durability in improving morbidity and mortality.
- Bariatric devices are a growing field of intervention that can further support patients in achieving their weight loss goals.

REFERENCES

1. National Heart, Lung, and Blood Institute Obesity Education Initiative Expert Panel on the Identification, Evaluation, and Treatment of Obesity in Adults (US). Clinical Guidelines on the Identification, Evaluation, and Treatment of Overweight and Obesity in Adults: The Evidence Report. Bethesda (MD): National Heart, Lung, and Blood Institute. 1998;98(4083):1–262.
2. Hales CM, Fryer CD, Ogden CL. Prevalence of obesity among adults and youth: United States, 2015-2016. Centers for Disease Control and Prevention; 2017. Available at: https://www.cdc.gov/nchs/products/databriefs/db288.htm. Accessed June 8, 2020.
3. Ward ZJ, Bleich SN, Cradock AL, et al. Projected U.S. state-level prevalence of adult obesity and severe obesity. N Engl J Med 2019;381(25):2440–50.
4. Garvey WT, Mechanick JI, Brett EM, et al. American Association of Clinical Endocrinologists and American College of Endocrinology comprehensive clinical practice guidelines for medical care of patients with obesity. Endocr Pract 2016;22(Suppl 3):1–203.
5. Jensen MD, Ryan DH, Apovian CM, et al. AHA/ACC/TOS Guideline for the management of overweight and obesity in adults: a report of the American College of Cardiology/American Heart Association/The Obesity Society Task Force on Practice Guidelines. J Am Coll Cardiol 2014;63(25 Pt B):2985–3023.
6. Heymsfield SB, Wadden TA. Mechanisms, pathophysiology, and management of obesity. N Engl J Med 2017;376(3):254–66.
7. Thaler JP, Yi CX, Schur EA, et al. Obesity is associated with hypothalamic injury in rodents and humans. J Clin Invest 2012;122(1):153–62.
8. Bays HE, Gonzalez-Campoy JM, Henry RR, et al. Is adiposopathy (sick fat) an endocrine disease? Int J Clin Pract 2008;62(10):1474–83.
9. Kushner RF, Batsis JA, Butsch WS, et al. Weight history in clinical practice: the state of the science and future directions. Obesity (Silver Spring) 2020; 28(1):9–17.

10. Pasquali R, Casanueva F, Haluzik M, et al. European Society of Endocrinology Clinical Practice Guideline: endocrine work-up in obesity. Eur J Endocrinol 2020;182(1):G1–32.

11. Apovian CM, Aronne LJ, Bessesen DH, et al. Pharmacological management of obesity: an endocrine society clinical practice guideline. J Clin Endocrinol Metab 2015;100(2):342–62.

12. World Health Organization. Appropriate body-mass index for Asian populations and its implications for policy and intervention strategies. Lancet 2004; 363(9403):157–63.

13. Trepanowski JF, Kroeger CM, Barnosky A, et al. Effect of alternate-day fasting on weight loss, weight maintenance, and cardioprotection among metabolically healthy obese adults: a randomized clinical trial. JAMA Intern Med 2017; 177(7):930–8.

14. Gabel K, Hoddy KK, Haggerty N, et al. Effects of 8-hour time restricted feeding on body weight and metabolic disease risk factors in obese adults: a pilot study. Nutr Healthy Aging 2018;4(4):345–53.

15. Knowler WC, Barrett-Connor E, Fowler SE, et al. Reduction in the incidence of type 2 diabetes with lifestyle intervention or metformin. N Engl J Med 2002; 346(6):393–403.

16. Pi-Sunyer X. The look AHEAD trial: a review and discussion of its outcomes. Curr Nutr Rep 2014;3(4):387–91.

17. Westman EC, Feinman RD, Mavropoulos JC, et al. Low-carbohydrate nutrition and metabolism. Am J Clin Nutr 2007;86(2):276–84.

18. Tobias DK, Chen M, Manson JE, et al. Effect of low-fat diet interventions versus other diet interventions on long-term weight change in adults: a systematic review and meta-analysis. Lancet Diabetes Endocrinol 2015;3(12):968–79.

19. Hu T, Mills KT, Yao L, et al. Effects of low-carbohydrate diets versus low-fat diets on metabolic risk factors: a meta-analysis of randomized controlled clinical trials. Am J Epidemiol 2012;176(Suppl 7):S44–54.

20. Bueno NB, de Melo IS, de Oliveira SL, et al. Very-low-carbohydrate ketogenic diet v. low-fat diet for long-term weight loss: a meta-analysis of randomised controlled trials. Br J Nutr 2013;110(7):1178–87.

21. Athinarayanan SJ, Adams RN, Hallberg SJ, et al. Long-term effects of a novel continuous remote care intervention including nutritional ketosis for the management of type 2 diabetes: a 2-year non-randomized clinical trial. Front Endocrinol (Lausanne) 2019;10:348.

22. Shai I, Schwarzfuchs D, Henkin Y, et al. Weight loss with a low-carbohydrate, Mediterranean, or low-fat diet. N Engl J Med 2008;359(3):229–41.

23. United States Department of Agriculture (USDA). ChooseMyPlate. USDA Center for Nutrition Policy & Promotion. 1994. Available at: www.choosemyplate.gov. Accessed March 11, 2020.

24. Dansinger ML, Gleason JA, Griffith JL, et al. Comparison of the Atkins, Ornish, Weight Watchers, and Zone diets for weight loss and heart disease risk reduction: a randomized trial. JAMA 2005;293(1):43–53.

25. Lopez-Minguez J, Gomez-Abellan P, Garaulet M. Timing of breakfast, lunch, and dinner. Effects on obesity and metabolic risk. Nutrients 2019;11(11):2624.

26. Jakubowicz D, Barnea M, Wainstein J, et al. High caloric intake at breakfast vs. dinner differentially influences weight loss of overweight and obese women. Obesity (Silver Spring) 2013;21(12):2504–12.

27. Lopez-Minguez J, Saxena R, Bandin C, et al. Late dinner impairs glucose tolerance in MTNR1B risk allele carriers: a randomized, cross-over study. Clin Nutr 2018;37(4):1133–40.

28. Bandin C, Scheer FA, Luque AJ, et al. Meal timing affects glucose tolerance, substrate oxidation and circadian-related variables: a randomized, crossover trial. Int J Obes (Lond) 2015;39(5):828–33.

29. Kant AK, Graubard BI. Within-person comparison of eating behaviors, time of eating, and dietary intake on days with and without breakfast: NHANES 2005-2010. Am J Clin Nutr 2015;102(3):661–70.

30. Donnelly JE, Blair SN, Jakicic JM, et al. American College of Sports Medicine Position Stand. Appropriate physical activity intervention strategies for weight loss and prevention of weight regain for adults. Med Sci Sports Exerc 2009;41(2): 459–71.

31. Donnelly JE, Hill JO, Jacobsen DJ, et al. Effects of a 16-month randomized controlled exercise trial on body weight and composition in young, overweight men and women: the Midwest Exercise Trial. Arch Intern Med 2003;163(11): 1343–50.

32. Fothergill E, Guo J, Howard L, et al. Persistent metabolic adaptation 6 years after "The Biggest Loser" competition. Obesity (Silver Spring) 2016;24(8):1612–9.

33. Pratley R, Nicklas B, Rubin M, et al. Strength training increases resting metabolic rate and norepinephrine levels in healthy 50- to 65-yr-old men. J Appl Physiol (1985) 1994;76(1):133–7.

34. Aristizabal JC, Freidenreich DJ, Volk BM, et al. Effect of resistance training on resting metabolic rate and its estimation by a dual-energy X-ray absorptiometry metabolic map. Eur J Clin Nutr 2015;69(7):831–6.

35. Wadden TA, Tronieri JS, Butryn ML. Lifestyle modification approaches for the treatment of obesity in adults. Am Psychol 2020;75(2):235–51.

36. Butryn ML, Webb V, Wadden TA. Behavioral treatment of obesity. Psychiatr Clin North Am 2011;34(4):841–59.

37. Klem ML, Wing RR, McGuire MT, et al. A descriptive study of individuals successful at long-term maintenance of substantial weight loss. Am J Clin Nutr 1997; 66(2):239–46.

38. Burke LE, Wang J, Sevick MA. Self-monitoring in weight loss: a systematic review of the literature. J Am Diet Assoc 2011;111(1):92–102.

39. Igel LI, Kumar RB, Saunders KH, et al. Practical use of pharmacotherapy for obesity. Gastroenterology 2017;152(7):1765–79.

40. Sumithran P, Prendergast LA, Delbridge E, et al. Long-term persistence of hormonal adaptations to weight loss. N Engl J Med 2011;365(17):1597–604.

41. Rothman RB, Baumann MH, Dersch CM, et al. Amphetamine-type central nervous system stimulants release norepinephrine more potently than they release dopamine and serotonin. Synapse 2001;39(1):32–41.

42. Kaplan LM. Pharmacological therapies for obesity. Gastroenterol Clin North Am 2005;34(1):91–104.

43. Aronne LJ, Wadden TA, Peterson C, et al. Evaluation of phentermine and topiramate versus phentermine/topiramate extended-release in obese adults. Obesity (Silver Spring) 2013;21(11):2163–71.

44. Genentech USA I. Xenical [Package Insert]. San Francisco, CA: Genentech USA, Inc; 2016.

45. Torgerson JS, Hauptman J, Boldrin MN, et al. XENical in the prevention of diabetes in obese subjects (XENDOS) study: a randomized study of orlistat as an

adjunct to lifestyle changes for the prevention of type 2 diabetes in obese patients. Diabetes Care 2004;27(1):155–61.

46. Allison DB, Gadde KM, Garvey WT, et al. Controlled-release phentermine/topiramate in severely obese adults: a randomized controlled trial (EQUIP). Obesity (Silver Spring) 2012;20(2):330–42.

47. Gadde KM, Allison DB, Ryan DH, et al. Effects of low-dose, controlled-release, phentermine plus topiramate combination on weight and associated comorbidities in overweight and obese adults (CONQUER): a randomised, placebo-controlled, phase 3 trial. Lancet 2011;377(9774):1341–52.

48. Garvey WT, Ryan DH, Look M, et al. Two-year sustained weight loss and metabolic benefits with controlled-release phentermine/topiramate in obese and overweight adults (SEQUEL): a randomized, placebo-controlled, phase 3 extension study. Am J Clin Nutr 2012;95(2):297–308.

49. Greenway FL, Whitehouse MJ, Guttadauria M, et al. Rational design of a combination medication for the treatment of obesity. Obesity (Silver Spring) 2009; 17(1):30–9.

50. Greenway FL, Fujioka K, Plodkowski RA, et al. Effect of naltrexone plus bupropion on weight loss in overweight and obese adults (COR-I): a multicentre, randomised, double-blind, placebo-controlled, phase 3 trial. Lancet 2010;376(9741): 595–605.

51. Apovian CM, Aronne L, Rubino D, et al. A randomized, phase 3 trial of naltrexone SR/bupropion SR on weight and obesity-related risk factors (COR-II). Obesity (Silver Spring) 2013;21(5):935–43.

52. Wadden TA, Foreyt JP, Foster GD, et al. Weight loss with naltrexone SR/bupropion SR combination therapy as an adjunct to behavior modification: the COR-BMOD trial. Obesity (Silver Spring) 2011;19(1):110–20.

53. Hollander P, Gupta AK, Plodkowski R, et al. Effects of naltrexone sustained-release/bupropion sustained-release combination therapy on body weight and glycemic parameters in overweight and obese patients with type 2 diabetes. Diabetes Care 2013;36(12):4022–9.

54. Nauck M, Frid A, Hermansen K, et al. Efficacy and safety comparison of liraglutide, glimepiride, and placebo, all in combination with metformin, in type 2 diabetes: the LEAD (liraglutide effect and action in diabetes)-2 study. Diabetes Care 2009;32(1):84–90.

55. van Can J, Sloth B, Jensen CB, et al. Effects of the once-daily GLP-1 analog liraglutide on gastric emptying, glycemic parameters, appetite and energy metabolism in obese, non-diabetic adults. Int J Obes (Lond) 2014;38(6):784–93.

56. Colquitt JL, Pickett K, Loveman E, et al. Surgery for weight loss in adults. Cochrane Database Syst Rev 2014;(8):CD003641.

57. American Society for Metabolic and Bariatric Surgery. Estimate of Bariatric Surgery Numbers, 2011-2018. ASMBS. 2018. Available at: https://asmbs.org/resources/estimate-of-bariatric-surgery-numbers. Accessed February 24, 2020.

58. Barenbaum SR, Saunders KH, Igel LI, et al. Obesity: when to consider surgery. J Fam Pract 2018;67(10):614, 616;618;620.

59. Courcoulas AP, King WC, Belle SH, et al. Seven-year weight trajectories and health outcomes in the Longitudinal Assessment of Bariatric Surgery (LABS) study. JAMA Surg 2018;153(5):427–34.

60. le Roux CW, Heneghan HM. Bariatric surgery for obesity. Med Clin North Am 2018;102(1):165–82.

61. Saunders KH, Igel LI, Saumoy M, et al. Devices and endoscopic bariatric therapies for obesity. Curr Obes Rep 2018;7(2):162–71.

62. Grundy SM, Cleeman JI, Daniels SR, et al. Diagnosis and management of the metabolic syndrome: an American Heart Association/National Heart, Lung, and Blood Institute Scientific Statement. Circulation 2005;112(17):2735–52.

63. Helfand M, Carson S. Screening for Lipid disorders in adults: selective Update of 2001 US preventive Services Task Force Review 2008. Rockville, MD.

64. Expert Panel on Detection, Evaluation, and Treatment of High Blood Cholesterol in Adults. Executive summary of the third report of the National Cholesterol Education Program (NCEP) expert panel on detection, evaluation, and treatment of high blood cholesterol in adults (adult treatment panel III). JAMA 2001;285(19):2486–97.

65. Selph S, Dana T, Blazina I, et al. Screening for type 2 diabetes mellitus: a systematic review for the U.S. Preventive Services Task Force. Ann Intern Med 2015;162(11):765–76.

66. American Diabetes Association. 2. Classification and diagnosis of diabetes. Diabetes Care 2020;43(Suppl 1):S14–31.

67. Harvie MN, Pegington M, Mattson MP, et al. The effects of intermittent or continuous energy restriction on weight loss and metabolic disease risk markers: a randomized trial in young overweight women. Int J Obes (Lond) 2011;35(5):714–27.

68. Longo VD, Panda S. Fasting, circadian rhythms, and time-restricted feeding in healthy lifespan. Cell Metab 2016;23(6):1048–59.

69. Orbera Intragastric Balloon [package insert]. Austin, TX: Apollo Endosurgery; 2015.

70. Courcoulas A, Abu Dayyeh BK, Eaton L, et al. Intragastric balloon as an adjunct to lifestyle intervention: a randomized controlled trial. Int J Obes (Lond) 2017;41(3):427–33.

71. U.S. Food and Drug Administration. PMA P140008: FDA summary of safety and effectiveness data. Available at: https://www.accessdata.fda.gov/cdrh_docs/pdf14/P140008b.pdf. Accessed February 24, 2020.

72. Obalon Balloon System [package insert]. Carlsbad, CA: Obalon Therapeutics, Inc; 2016.

73. Sullivan S, Swain JM, Woodman G, et al. The Obalon Swallowable 6-Month Balloon System is More Effective Than Moderate Intensity Lifestyle Therapy Alone: Results From a 6- Month Randomized Sham Controlled Trial. Gastroenterology 2016;150(4):S1267.

74. U.S. Food and Drug Administration. PMA P160001: FDA summary of safety and effectiveness data. Available at: https://www.accessdata.fda.gov/cdrh_docs/pdf16/P160001b.pdf. Accessed February 24, 2020.

75. AspireAssist [package insert]. King of Prussia, PA: Aspire Bariatrics; 2016.

76. Thompson CC, Dayyeh BKA, Kushner R, et al. The AspireAssist is an effective tool in the treatment of class II and class III obesity: results of a one-year clinical trial. Gastroenterology 2016;150(4):S86.

77. Gelesis Inc. Plenity [package insert]. Boston: Gelesis, Inc; 2019.

78. Greenway FL, Aronne LJ, Raben A, et al. A randomized, double-blind, placebo-controlled study of Gelesis100: a novel nonsystemic oral hydrogel for weight loss. Obesity (Silver Spring) 2019;27(2):205–16.

79. TransPyloric Shuttle [package insert]. San Carlos, CA: BAROnova, Inc; 2019.

80. U.S. Food and Drug Administration. PMA P180024: FDA summary of safety and effectiveness data. Available at: https://www.accessdata.fda.gov/cdrh_docs/pdf18/P180024B.pdf. Accessed February 24, 2020.

Approach to Patients with Unintentional Weight Loss

Liyanage Ashanthi Menaka Perera, MD[a,1], Aparna Chopra, MBBS[b,1], Amy L. Shaw, MD[c,*]

KEYWORDS

- Weight loss • Unintentional weight loss • Involuntary weight loss
- Unintended weight loss • Malignancy • Older adults

KEY POINTS

- Unintentional weight loss is a common problem, especially in older adults, and is associated with increased mortality.
- The most common causes are malignancy, nonmalignant gastrointestinal diseases, and psychiatric disorders in community-dwelling adults; psychiatric disorders are the most common cause identified in institutionalized older adults.
- Treatment of unintentional weight loss is aimed at managing the underlying causes.

INTRODUCTION

Unintentional weight loss can be an enigma for internists. It is a nonspecific condition that may come to light either through the observations of a discerning family member or physician or as a chief complaint from the patient themselves. The differential diagnosis is broad, and the clinician is then faced with the task of ascertaining how and where to begin the search for a cause. In this review, the authors aim to summarize the potential causes of unintentional weight loss and review treatment options. They also offer insight into the management of unintentional weight loss in older adults.

In the literature, unintentional weight loss is used synonymously with "involuntary" or "unintended" weight loss. It is used to describe situations whereby weight loss occurs without effort on the part of the patient and whereby it is not an expected consequence of the treatment of a known medical condition or illness, such as diuretic

[a] Department of Medicine, Division of Hospital Internal Medicine, Mayo Clinic, 1000 First Drive NW, Austin, Minnesota, 55912, USA; [b] Institute for Critical Care Medicine, The Mount Sinai Hospital, 1468 Madison Avenue, Guggenheim Pavilion 6 East, Room 378, New York, New York, USA; [c] Department of Medicine, Division of Geriatrics and Palliative Medicine, Weill Cornell Medicine, 525 East 68th Street, Box 39, New York, NY 10065, USA
[1] Co-first author.
* Corresponding author.
E-mail address: als9138@med.cornell.edu
Twitter: @amyshawmd (A.L.S.)

Med Clin N Am 105 (2021) 175–186
https://doi.org/10.1016/j.mcna.2020.08.019
0025-7125/21/© 2020 Elsevier Inc. All rights reserved.

therapy for heart failure exacerbation. Furthermore, unintentional weight loss is not synonymous with other wasting disorders, such as sarcopenia or cachexia. Sarcopenia is a multifaceted geriatric syndrome characterized by progressive loss of skeletal muscle mass and strength; it is attributed to primary (age-related) or secondary (multimorbidity-related) causes, and it is often associated with debility, poor quality of life, and death.[1] Cachexia, on the other hand, describes muscle loss in the setting of underlying illness, often associated with anorexia, inflammation, and insulin resistance.[2,3] Although these conditions are not synonymous with unintentional weight loss, patients may develop both sarcopenia and cachexia as a result of their weight loss.

NATURE OF THE PROBLEM

Several large studies have shown an association between unintentional weight loss and mortality in specific populations, including American women aged 55 to 69,[4] British men aged 56 to 75,[5] and overweight and obese American people aged 35 and over.[6]

The connection between unintentional weight loss and mortality is especially important given that unintentional weight loss is not uncommon. One large survey study among people 45 years of age and older found that 5% of participants reported unintentional weight loss of at least 5% in the preceding 12 months; unintentional weight loss was associated with older age, smoking, and poorer health status.[7] In the longer term, approximately 15% to 20% of people 65 years of age and older are estimated to develop unintentional weight loss over 5 to 10 years.[8]

DEFINITIONS

Beginning in the third decade of life, physiologic changes to body mass composition as a result of the normal process of aging leads to lean body mass decline at a rate of 0.3 kg/y with a simultaneous increase in body fat. The net result of these changes is an increase in total body weight that peaks in the fifth to sixth decade of life, with weight remaining stable until age 65 to 70.[9] By the seventh decade, patients begin to lose weight at a rate of 0.1 to 0.2 kg/y; unintentional weight loss exceeding these parameters is considered abnormal.[10] Although there is not yet a consensus on what constitutes clinically significant weight loss, many studies in the literature have used a cutoff of 5% loss of usual body weight over a span of 6 to 12 months as the definition of clinically significant weight loss warranting further medical evaluation.[11]

PATHOPHYSIOLOGY

Cancer cachexia may provide insight into the biological mechanisms behind unintentional weight loss. The proinflammatory cytokines, tumor necrosis factor alpha, interleukin-1, and interleukin-6, are implicated in driving cancer cachexia by promoting anorexia as well as muscle and fat catabolism.[12]

In order to maintain body weight homeostasis, energy intake must be equivalent to energy expenditure. In cancer cachexia, however, the decreased caloric intake does not result in decreased energy expenditure[12]; rather, it is a hypermetabolic state with an upregulation in the biochemical processes of gluconeogenesis, protein breakdown, lipolysis,[13] and lactate recycling.[12] For example, resting energy expenditure has been shown to be elevated in patients with lung cancer, and higher resting energy expenditure is correlated with higher levels of the inflammatory marker C-reactive protein.[14] Leptin, a hormone produced by adipocytes, acts upon the receptors of the hypothalamus to produce a negative feedback mechanism that results in satiety and decreased food intake. Although patients with caloric deprivation and those with cancer cachexia have low leptin levels, patients with cancer cachexia do not have the normal resulting increase in appetite and decrease in energy expenditure; inflammation is thought to interfere with the normal feedback system.[15] The metabolic, hormonal, and cytokine dysregulation seen in cancer cachexia demonstrates the complexity of the mechanisms that potentially lie behind undifferentiated unintentional weight loss.

CAUSES OF UNINTENTIONAL WEIGHT LOSS

Unintentional weight loss is a marker for serious underlying pathologic condition. Several studies that investigated causes of unintentional weight loss found that malignancy is the most common cause, found in 15% to 37% of patients.[16–18] Nonmalignant gastrointestinal causes (particularly malabsorption disorders) constitute 10% to 20% of cases,[17–20] whereas psychiatric disorders (particularly depression) make up another 10% to 23% of cases of unintentional weight loss.[16–18] Surprisingly, another 25% of cases do not find a cause for unintentional weight loss despite a thorough workup.[16,17] It is important to note that many studies describing the causes of unintentional weight loss have been conducted at referral centers after some initial workup was unrevealing, so the true distribution of causes in primary care may be different. In other words, studies from referral centers may reflect the causes that are found after the most common causes have been elicited in primary care. It is also important to note that advances in imaging and other medical technology may reduce the proportion of patients with idiopathic weight loss in current practice compared with the proportion of these patients in older studies. Conditions to consider in the differential diagnosis of unintentional weight loss are described in detail in later discussion.

Malignancy

Malignancies are associated with anorexia and weight loss at the time of diagnosis, particularly upper gastrointestinal cancer (80%) and lung cancer (60%).[21] Workup for weight loss associated with malignancy may require additional testing. In a prospective cohort study conducted by Metalidis and colleagues,[22] among 101 patients, all 22 patients who had an underlying malignancy had abnormal laboratory test results, including C-reactive protein, hemoglobin, lactate dehydrogenase, and albumin. However, imaging studies, such as ultrasound and chest radiographs, had lower sensitivities (45% and 18%, respectively).

Cardiovascular Disease

Congestive heart failure can lead to both sarcopenia and cachexia, although edema may mask the diagnosis of weight loss.[23] Cachexia predicts mortality in heart failure independent of factors, such as age, New York Heart Association symptom class, and left ventricular ejection fraction.[23] Various factors have been implicated in the pathophysiology of cardiac cachexia, which involves alterations in energy expenditure and catabolic-anabolic balance. These factors include both increased production of the proinflammatory cytokines, interleukin-1, interleukin-6, and tumor necrosis factor alpha, and increased sympathetic nervous system activity with resulting stimulation of the renin-angiotensin-aldosterone system.[24]

Respiratory Disease

Chronic weight loss that is associated with severe lung disease is called pulmonary cachexia syndrome. Approximately 25% of patients with chronic obstructive pulmonary disease are estimated to develop cachexia; the pathophysiology of weight loss is likely related to disuse atrophy, tissue hypoxia, systemic inflammation, and neurohormonal dysregulation, including insufficiency of anabolic hormones and sympathetic upregulation.[25] The pattern of weight loss is frequently episodic, with a decline associated with each acute exacerbation. Glucocorticoid treatment may compound the loss of lean body mass.[26] Other pulmonary conditions associated with unintentional weight loss may overlap with inflammatory (eg, interstitial lung disease and ANCA-associated vasculitis), infectious (eg, tuberculous and nontuberculous mycobacterial infections), and malignant (eg, lung cancer) conditions, illustrating that causes of weight loss commonly involve more than 1 body system.

Gastrointestinal Disease

A thorough history and physical examination may reveal symptoms suggestive of gastrointestinal disease. These clinical features include abdominal pain, early satiety, dysphagia, odynophagia, steatorrhea, hematochezia, melena, abdominal tenderness, and abdominal masses. Although gastrointestinal malignancy, inflammatory bowel disease, and malabsorption (eg, pancreatic insufficiency and celiac sprue) are commonly thought of as gastrointestinal causes of weight loss, clinicians should also consider conditions such as peptic ulcer disease, mesenteric ischemia, and protein-losing enteropathies.[26] The mouth and pharynx are important parts of the gastrointestinal tract, and mechanical difficulties, such as dysphagia, odynophagia, and poor dentition, from any cause may contribute to weight loss by affecting the desire or ability to chew and swallow food.[27]

Endocrinopathies

Hyperthyroidism is associated with accelerated weight loss and increased appetite.[28] Patients with uncontrolled diabetes mellitus may experience weight loss along with other symptoms of hyperglycemia, such as polyuria and polydipsia.[29] Primary adrenal insufficiency may present with the nonspecific symptoms of weight loss, nausea, and fatigue.[30]

Rheumatologic Disease

Unintentional weight loss may be a presenting symptom in certain rheumatological conditions, particularly rheumatoid arthritis, where the term "rheumatoid cachexia" describes a loss of skeletal muscle and gain of fat mass.[31] Giant cell arteritis may also be associated with weight loss,[32,33] as may autoimmune and inflammatory conditions mentioned elsewhere, such as inflammatory bowel disease and ANCA-associated vasculitis.

Infectious Disease

AIDS can lead to episodic weight loss related to secondary opportunistic infections, low CD4 count states, and malabsorptive gastrointestinal diseases. The mechanism for weight loss is multifactorial but primarily related to increased energy expenditure during opportunistic infections and excessive cytokine activation states coupled with reduced oral intake that leads to protein-calorie malnutrition resembling wasting and starvation.[34–36] Other infectious diseases, such as active and reactivation tuberculosis, chronic hepatitis C, and helminthic infections, can commonly present with weight loss. Clinicians should consider local disease patterns and patient travel history when investigating possible infectious disease.

Neurodegenerative and Psychiatric Disease

Weight loss is commonly seen in neurodegenerative diseases, such as Alzheimer-type dementia, Parkinson disease, and Huntington disease; in Alzheimer disease and Parkinson disease, weight loss may precede diagnosis.[37,38] Related cognitive impairment may cause difficulty remembering to eat or preparing food. Psychiatric disorders, particularly depression, are a common cause of unintentional weight loss. A prospective study of 2677 patients with unintentional weight loss found 16% of cases were the result of psychiatric conditions.[16] The proportion of people with unintentional weight loss attributed to psychiatric causes can exceed 50% in nursing home residents.[16,39,40] Patients of all ages, genders, and races may suffer from eating disorders; patients with eating disorders may present to primary care with a variety of concerns before an eating disorder is diagnosed.[41]

Medications and Substances

Weight loss is a common adverse effect of many medications. Anticonvulsants (topiramate), antidepressants (bupropion), and stimulants eg. methylphenidate, dextroamphetamine can cause weight loss as a result of appetite suppression. Other classes of medications can lead to unintentional weight loss as a result of decreased oral intake from medication-induced nausea and vomiting (selective serotonin reuptake inhibitors, tricyclic antidepressants, dopamine agonists, metformin, digoxin), alterations in taste and smell (angiotensin converting enzyme inhibitors, calcium channel blockers, spironolactone, allopurinol), and dry mouth (anticholinergic medications). Dysphagia as a result of pill esophagitis from medications, such as bisphosphonates, doxycycline, potassium supplements, and nonsteroidal anti-inflammatory drugs, can also limit oral intake. Gastrointestinal symptoms, such as diarrhea, potentiate the effect of weight loss and are a commonly experienced adverse effect of medications, such as metformin, glucagon-like peptide-1 agonists, and laxatives.[8,11,42]

In addition to prescribed medications, other substances can also lead to weight loss. Although the mechanism is still unclear, cocaine is thought to cause weight loss in part through appetite suppression as well as by dysregulation of fat metabolism leading to reduction in fat body mass.[43] Amphetamines and their stimulant derivatives cause weight loss through appetite suppression and increased energy expenditure. Excess alcohol consumption and dependence can lead to a nutrition-deficient diet of "empty calories" leading to malnutrition and subsequently weight loss.

Clinicians must gather a complete history of all medications and substances taken by patients, being aware that patients may obtain prescription drugs from other clinicians or from other people (ie, by using a prescription written for someone else) and may use over-the-counter medications or supplements that can contribute to weight loss.

Psychosocial Factors

Social determinants of health, such as socioeconomic status, physical environment, and social support networks, can affect access to food, leading to unintentional weight loss. Patients with functional or cognitive impairment may have difficulty performing tasks, such as grocery shopping and preparing food. Clinicians should be aware that older adults, especially those with cognitive impairment who depend on caregivers, are at increased risk for elder abuse and neglect.

CAUSES OF WEIGHT LOSS IN OLDER ADULTS

Unintentional weight loss is common in older adults and occurs in about 15% to 20% of geriatric patients.[44] It is even more prevalent in high-risk populations, such as nursing home residents, with estimates of up to 60%.[45] Unintentional weight loss in older adults is associated with an increased risk of mortality even when controlling for potential confounders like smoking and alcohol use,[46] sedentariness,[44] and comorbidities.[44,46,47] It is also associated with a decline in activities of daily living,[44,48] decreased quality of life,[49] increased risk of hip fractures,[50] and increased hospital length of stay and complications.[51] Unintentional weight loss in older adults is even associated with subsequent admission to long-term care institutions.[52] Risk factors for unintentional weight loss in this patient population include presence of comorbidities, low body weight, smoking, low education level, loss of a spouse,[7] and cognitive impairment.[38]

The causes of unintentional weight loss in older adults are similar to the causes of unintentional weight loss in the general population, with malignancy being the most common cause (16% to 36%), followed by nonmalignant gastrointestinal diseases (10% to 20%) and psychiatric disorders, such as depression or dementia (10% to 23%), in community-dwelling older adults.[16,17,19,42,53] In long-term care facilities, psychiatric disorders are the most common cause of unintentional weight loss.[40]

Unlike their younger counterparts, older adults more often have multiple causes of unintentional weight loss related to the physiology of aging and the interplay of chronic medical conditions. Older adults may have decreased appetite as a result of decreased energy requirements, due in part to decreases in lean muscle mass and increases in total body fat. However, this becomes pathologic when the degree of loss of appetite becomes disproportionately higher than the reduction in energy expenditure, and subsequently, weight loss exceeds the expected small loss in weight with age.[54] Physiologic changes related to aging, such as decreased taste and olfactory sensation and slower gastric emptying coupled with early satiation, contribute to reduced pleasure or interest in eating and predispose older adults to weight loss.[55] The presence of oropharyngeal and esophageal disorders related to dental decay, dry mouth, and dysphagia can potentiate this effect and further precipitate weight loss. Polypharmacy can alter taste-smell sensorium and can increase the likelihood of anorexia-related adverse effects of medications. Furthermore, socioeconomic constraints, such as limitations in obtaining and preparing food, may be significant, especially in frail, socially isolated older adults.

APPROACH

The workup of unintentional weight loss relies on a thorough history and physical examination to diagnose disease and guide testing (**Fig. 1**). A clinical history should include the amount and pace of weight loss; dietary assessment; psychosocial factors; and associated symptoms, such as joint pain, dyspnea, diarrhea, gastrointestinal bleeding, dental problems, and depressed mood. Clinicians should review all medications, supplements, and chronic medical conditions. A physical examination can reveal signs of weight loss, such as temporal wasting and loose clothing. It can also reveal signs of serious illness, such as lymphadenopathy, joint swelling, cardiopulmonary abnormalities, organomegaly, and masses (eg, on prostate, breast, and abdominal examination). Oral examination may show poor dentition or painful lesions, and cognitive screening may alert clinicians to impairment.[11,26,56]

The authors suggest that the initial laboratory, radiologic, and other testing be guided by the results of the history and physical examination. For example, endoscopy would be considered early in the workup of a patient with weight loss, melena, abdominal pain, and early satiety but would not be part of the initial evaluation for weight loss in general. Laboratory tests to consider include a complete blood count

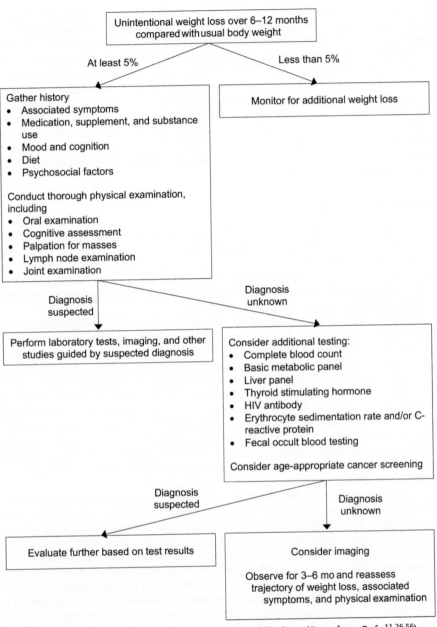

Fig. 1. Suggested initial workup of unintentional weight loss. (*Data from* Refs.[11,26,56])

to look for infection, anemia, and lymphoproliferative disorders; a comprehensive metabolic panel to look for diabetes, liver disease, renal insufficiency, and electrolyte abnormalities; a thyroid function profile to rule out hyperthyroidism; lactate dehydrogenase, which may be elevated in malignancy; inflammatory markers, such as erythrocyte sedimentation rate and C-reactive protein, which may be elevated in inflammatory, malignant, or infectious conditions; and tests for HIV and chronic viral hepatitis. Testing for chronic viral hepatitis should be considered based on risk factors. One-time fecal occult blood testing is often used to screen for colon cancer but is neither sensitive nor specific; a negative result does not rule out bleeding or malignancy, so diagnostic studies, such as endoscopy and colonoscopy, may become necessary if there is suspicion for gastrointestinal malignancy or inflammatory conditions. Imaging studies, such as computed tomography, may be pursued if indicated based on the history, physical examination, and initial tests.[11,56] Age-appropriate cancer screening should be pursued if it is not up-to-date.

If this workup reveals abnormal results suggestive of a particular cause of the unintentional weight loss, then a targeted evaluation and treatment of the underlying cause are indicated. If these studies are uniformly normal, then the patient should be monitored over the next 3 to 6 months to look for additional weight loss or signs and symptoms to guide further workup.

THERAPEUTIC OPTIONS

Treatment of patients with unintentional weight loss involves treating the underlying cause. A thorough history and physical examination are vital in order to identify the cause of weight loss and can be supplemented by laboratory tests as well as age-appropriate cancer screening. An interprofessional approach, including dietitians, speech therapists (for evaluation of oropharyngeal dysphagia), and social services, is imperative in treating unintentional weight loss.[40]

Several medications, most commonly mirtazapine, dronabinol, and megestrol, have been used to promote weight gain, although side effects may limit their use. These medications have also not been shown to improve mortality in older adults with unintentional weight loss.[8,11] Mirtazapine, a selective serotonin reuptake inhibitor, may be used to treat patients with depression who have reduced appetite; treatment improves appetite and promotes weight gain, but adverse effects include dry mouth, dizziness, orthostatic hypotension, and excessive sedation.[11,57] Dronabinol, a cannabinoid, has been used for the treatment of anorexia in patients with AIDS but can have central nervous system toxicity, including confusion and somnolence.[11,40] Although megestrol has been found to improve appetite and promote weight gain in patients with cancer and patients with AIDS-related anorexia-cachexia syndrome, it is also associated with adverse effects, such as edema, thromboembolic events, and death.[58]

In older adults, altering the consistency of food can help accommodate patients with poor dentition or dysphagia. Reducing dietary restrictions, such as low-fat or low-salt diets, may be appropriate to make food more palatable. Nutritional supplements can provide extra calories but should not replace meals; they may be more effective when given between meals.[59] Weight loss refractory to oral nutritional supplementation may elicit questions from patients, families, and clinicians about feeding tube placement. This discussion must incorporate patient and caregiver preferences as well as acknowledgments of risks and benefits of tube feeding.[40] Tube feeding is associated with higher mortality in nursing home residents with dysphagia compared with residents without tube feeding, even when adjusted for factors such as weight loss and pressure injury.[60] Feeding tubes may need to be replaced or repositioned.[61] Furthermore, percutaneous endoscopic gastrostomy tube placement improves neither mortality nor albumin levels in patients with dementia compared with patients having PEG placement for other neurologic diseases or head and neck cancers.[62] It should be noted that decision-making about tube feeding in nursing home patients and patients with dementia may differ from decision-making about tube feeding in patients with other conditions, especially those whose underlying condition is expected to improve.[60]

SUMMARY

Clinically significant weight loss is defined as a loss of at least 5% of body weight over 6 to 12 months. There is an increase in morbidity and mortality associated with unintentional weight loss. The differential diagnosis of involuntary weight loss is broad and requires consideration of physiologic, pathologic, and psychosocial factors. Treatment largely depends on targeting the underlying cause; therefore, clinicians must perform a thorough history and physical examination and consider laboratory testing and cancer screening when evaluating a patient with unintentional weight loss.

CLINICS CARE POINTS

- Many studies define clinically significant weight loss as at least 5% of usual body weight over 6 to 12 months (source 11).
- Weight loss is associated with many chronic diseases.
- A careful medication history is essential in the workup of weight loss; medications may lead to weight loss through several mechanisms.
- Nutritional supplements should be used to supplement rather than replace regular meals (source 59).

DISCLOSURE

Dr. Shaw supported in part by a Joachim Silbermann Family Clinical Scholar Award in Geriatrics from the Rosanne H. Silbermann Foundation.

REFERENCES

1. Santilli V, Bernetti A, Mangone M, et al. Clinical definition of sarcopenia. Clin Cases Miner Bone Metab 2014;11:177–80.
2. Argilés JM, López-Soriano FJ, Toledo M, et al. The cachexia score (CASCO): a new tool for staging cachectic cancer patients. J Cachexia Sarcopenia Muscle 2011;2:87–93.
3. Evans WJ, Morley JE, Argilés J, et al. Cachexia: a new definition. Clin Nutr 2008; 27:793–9.
4. French SA, Folsom AR, Jeffery RW, et al. Prospective study of intentionality of weight loss and mortality in older women: the Iowa Women's Health Study. Am J Epidemiol 1999;149:504–14.
5. Wannamethee SG, Shaper AG, Lennon L. Reasons for intentional weight loss, unintentional weight loss, and mortality in older men. Arch Intern Med 2005;165: 1035–40.
6. Gregg EW, Gerzoff RB, Thompson TJ, et al. Intentional weight loss and death in overweight and obese U.S. adults 35 years of age and older. Ann Intern Med 2003;138:383–9.
7. Meltzer AA, Everhart JE. Unintentional weight loss in the United States. Am J Epidemiol 1995;142:1039–46.
8. Alibhai SMH, Greenwood C, Payette H. An approach to the management of unintentional weight loss in elderly people. Can Med Assoc J 2005;172:773–80.
9. Kuczmarski RJ. Need for body composition information in elderly subjects. Am J Clin Nutr 1989;50:1150–7.
10. Chumlea WC, Rhyne RL, Garry PJ, et al. Changes in anthropometric indices of body composition with age in a healthy elderly population. Am J Hum Biol 1989;1:457–62.

11. Gaddey HL, Holder K. Unintentional weight loss in older adults. Am Fam Physician 2014;89:718–22.

12. Argilés JM, Busquets S, Felipe A, et al. Molecular mechanisms involved in muscle wasting in cancer and ageing: cachexia versus sarcopenia. Int J Biochem Cell Biol 2005;37:1084–104.

13. Fearon KCH, Glass DJ, Guttridge DC. Cancer cachexia: mediators, signaling, and metabolic pathways. Cell Metab 2012;16:153–66.

14. Staal-van den Brekel AJ, Schols AM, ten Velde GP, et al. Analysis of the energy balance in lung cancer patients. Cancer Res 1994;54:6430–3.

15. Engineer DR, Garcia JM. Leptin in anorexia and cachexia syndrome. Int J Pept 2012;2012:287457.

16. Bosch X, Monclús E, Escoda O, et al. Unintentional weight loss: clinical characteristics and outcomes in a prospective cohort of 2677 patients. PLoS One 2017; 12:e0175125.

17. Rabinovitz M, Pitlik SD, Leifer M, et al. Unintentional weight loss. A retrospective analysis of 154 cases. Arch Intern Med 1986;146:186–7.

18. Hernández JL, Riancho JA, Matorras P, et al. Clinical evaluation for cancer in patients with involuntary weight loss without specific symptoms. Am J Med 2003; 114:631–7.

19. Marton KI, Sox HC, Krupp JR. Involuntary weight loss: diagnostic and prognostic significance. Ann Intern Med 1981;95:568–74.

20. Lankisch P, Gerzmann M, Gerzmann JF, et al. Unintentional weight loss: diagnosis and prognosis. The first prospective follow-up study from a secondary referral centre. J Intern Med 2001;249:41–6.

21. Inui A. Cancer anorexia-cachexia syndrome: current issues in research and management. CA Cancer J Clin 2002;52:72–91.

22. Metalidis C, Knockaert DC, Bobbaers H, et al. Involuntary weight loss. Does a negative baseline evaluation provide adequate reassurance? Eur J Intern Med 2008;19:345–9.

23. von Haehling S, Ebner N, Dos Santos MR, et al. Muscle wasting and cachexia in heart failure: mechanisms and therapies. Nat Rev Cardiol 2017;14:323–41.

24. Martins T, Vitorino R, Moreira-Gonçalves D, et al. Recent insights on the molecular mechanisms and therapeutic approaches for cardiac cachexia. Clin Biochem 2014;47:8–15.

25. Wagner PD. Possible mechanisms underlying the development of cachexia in COPD. Eur Respir J 2008;31:492–501.

26. Wong CJ. Involuntary weight loss. Med Clin North Am 2014;98:625–43.

27. Sullivan DH, Martin W, Flaxman N, et al. Oral health problems and involuntary weight loss in a population of frail elderly. J Am Geriatr Soc 1993;41:725–31.

28. Nordyke RA, Gilbert FI, Harada AS. Graves' disease. Influence of age on clinical findings. Arch Intern Med 1988;148:626–31.

29. American Diabetes Association. Diagnosis and classification of diabetes mellitus. Diabetes Care 2011;34(suppl 1):S62–9.

30. Erichsen MM, Løvås K, Skinningsrud B, et al. Clinical, immunological, and genetic features of autoimmune primary adrenal insufficiency: observations from a Norwegian registry. J Clin Endocrinol Metab 2009;94:4882–90.

31. Roubenoff R. Rheumatoid cachexia: a complication of rheumatoid arthritis moves into the 21st century. Arthritis Res Ther 2009;11:108.

32. Kapadia A, Abu J, Deen S, et al. An unusual case of abdominal pain and weight loss. Rheumatology (Oxford) 2020;59(8):2185–6.

33. Shukla S, Hull R. Think of giant cell arteritis. BMJ 2011;342:d2889.

34. Williams B, Waters D, Parker K. Evaluation and treatment of weight loss in adults with HIV disease. Am Fam Physician 1999;60:843–54, 857.

35. Grinspoon S, Mulligan K, Department of Health and Human Services Working Group on the Prevention and Treatment of Wasting and Weight Loss. Weight loss and wasting in patients infected with human immunodeficiency virus. Clin Infect Dis 2003;36:S69–78.

36. Mangili A, Murman DH, Zampini AM, et al. Nutrition and HIV infection: review of weight loss and wasting in the era of highly active antiretroviral therapy from the nutrition for healthy living cohort. Clin Infect Dis 2006;42:836–42.

37. Aziz NA, van der Marck MA, Pijl H, et al. Weight loss in neurodegenerative disorders. J Neurol 2008;255:1872–80.

38. Barrett-Connor E, Edelstein SL, Corey-Bloom J, et al. Weight loss precedes dementia in community-dwelling older adults. J Am Geriatr Soc 1996;44:1147–52.

39. Morley JE, Kraenzle D. Causes of weight loss in a community nursing home. J Am Geriatr Soc 1994;42:583–5.

40. Huffman GB. Evaluating and treating unintentional weight loss in the elderly. Am Fam Physician 2002;65:640–50.

41. Ogg EC, Millar HR, Pusztai EE, et al. General practice consultation patterns preceding diagnosis of eating disorders. Int J Eat Disord 1997;22:89–93.

42. Stajkovic S, Aitken EM, Holroyd-Leduc J. Unintentional weight loss in older adults. Can Med Assoc J 2011;183:443–9.

43. Ersche KD, Stochl J, Woodward JM, et al. The skinny on cocaine: insights into eating behavior and body weight in cocaine-dependent men. Appetite 2013;71:75–80.

44. Newman AB, Yanez D, Harris T, et al. Weight change in old age and its association with mortality. J Am Geriatr Soc 2001;49:1309–18.

45. Sullivan DH, Johnson LE, Bopp MM, et al. Prognostic significance of monthly weight fluctuations among older nursing home residents. J Gerontol A Biol Sci Med Sci 2004;59:M633–9.

46. Payette H, Coulombe C, Boutier V, et al. Weight loss and mortality among free-living frail elders: a prospective study. J Gerontol A Biol Sci Med Sci 1999;54:M440–5.

47. Somes GW, Kritchevsky SB, Shorr RI, et al. Body mass index, weight change, and death in older adults: the systolic hypertension in the elderly program. Am J Epidemiol 2002;156:132–8.

48. Launer LJ, Harris T, Rumpel C, et al. Body mass index, weight change, and risk of mobility disability in middle-aged and older women. The epidemiologic follow-up study of NHANES I. JAMA 1994;271:1093–8.

49. Fine JT, Colditz GA, Coakley EH, et al. A prospective study of weight change and health-related quality of life in women. JAMA 1999;282:2136–42.

50. Ensrud KE, Ewing SK, Stone KL, et al. Intentional and unintentional weight loss increase bone loss and hip fracture risk in older women. J Am Geriatr Soc 2003;51:1740–7.

51. Satish S, Winograd CH, Chavez C, et al. Geriatric targeting criteria as predictors of survival and health care utilization. J Am Geriatr Soc 1996;44:914–21.

52. Payette H, Coulombe C, Boutier V, et al. Nutrition risk factors for institutionalization in a free-living functionally dependent elderly population. J Clin Epidemiol 2000;53:579–87.

53. Vanderschueren S, Geens E, Knockaert D, et al. The diagnostic spectrum of unintentional weight loss. Eur J Intern Med 2005;16:160–4.

54. Wysokiński A, Sobów T, Kłoszewska I, et al. Mechanisms of the anorexia of aging—a review. Age (Dordr) 2015;37:9821.
55. Morley JE. Decreased food intake with aging. J Gerontol A Biol Sci Med Sci 2001; 56(2, special issue):81–8.
56. McMinn J, Steel C, Bowman A. Investigation and management of unintentional weight loss in older adults. BMJ 2011;342:d1732.
57. Fawcett J, Barkin RL. Review of the results from clinical studies on the efficacy, safety and tolerability of mirtazapine for the treatment of patients with major depression. J Affect Disord 1998;51:267–85.
58. Ruiz Garcia V, López-Briz E, Carbonell Sanchis R, et al. Megestrol acetate for treatment of anorexia-cachexia syndrome. Cochrane Database Syst Rev 2013;(3):CD004310.
59. Padala KP, Keller BK, Potter JF. Weight loss treatment in long-term care. J Nutr Elder 2008;26:1–20.
60. Mitchell SL, Kiely DK, Lipsitz LA. Does artificial enteral nutrition prolong the survival of institutionalized elders with chewing and swallowing problems? J Gerontol A Biol Sci Med Sci 1998;53:M207–13.
61. Kuo S, Rhodes RL, Mitchell SL, et al. Natural history of feeding-tube use in nursing home residents with advanced dementia. J Am Med Dir Assoc 2009; 10:264–70.
62. Ayman AR, Khoury T, Cohen J, et al. PEG insertion in patients with dementia does not improve nutritional status and has worse outcomes as compared with PEG insertion for other indications. J Clin Gastroenterol 2017;51:417–20.

Common Complaints of the Hands and Feet

David Jacob Aizenberg, MD

KEYWORDS

- Osteoarthritis • Carpal tunnel syndrome • Ganglion cyst • Plantar fasciitis
- Onychomycosis • Morton neuroma

KEY POINTS

- This article describes the typical presentations of 3 common diagnoses of the hands and 3 common diagnoses of the feet.
- Emphasis is placed on describing pearls that can be elucidated in the history and examination.
- Treatments that can be initiated without a referral to a specialist are reviewed.

 Video content accompanies this article at http://www.medical.theclinics.com.

INTRODUCTION

Humans constantly use their hands and feet in their daily life. When there is an abnormality in their function, it can cause significant distress. Primary care physicians frequently see these complaints in their offices. This article reviews some of the more common ailments with high-yield clinical care points that will help providers in general practice identify, examine, and treat these conditions.

HAND OSTEOARTHRITIS
Background

Hand osteoarthritis (OA) is a highly prevalent condition that can affect multiple joints. It impacts quality of life for a significant portion of the population.[1] It is more common in women than men and increases in prevalence with age. Once recognized, progression is typically slow but can be debilitating. Hand OA is a degenerative disease of the joints, and the role of inflammation continues to be contentious.[1]

Department of Medicine, Perelman School of Medicine at the University of Pennsylvania, 3701 Market Street, 7th Floor, Philadelphia, PA 19104, USA
E-mail address: david.aizenberg@pennmedicine.upenn.edu
Twitter: @daveaizenberg (D.J.A.)

Med Clin N Am 105 (2021) 187–197
https://doi.org/10.1016/j.mcna.2020.08.016
0025-7125/21/© 2020 Elsevier Inc. All rights reserved.

Clinical Features

Symptoms of hand OA usually include pain, stiffness, and decreased range of motion. Although heterogeneous, hand OA typically involves the carpometacarpal joint of the thumb. Firm nodules and swelling over the dorsal aspects of distal interphalangeal joints (Heberden nodes) or proximal interphalangeal joints (Bouchard nodes) are commonly found in patients with hand OA.[1]

Patients frequently report pain at the base of the thumb that usually worsens with activity. As the disease progresses, it becomes painful to open jars, twist doorknobs, or perform fine-motor activities. Patients can also lose grip strength.[2] Patients with prominent Bouchard or Heberden nodes may report pain at those sites and frequently complain of aesthetic dissatisfaction with the appearance of their hands.

Physical Examination

Findings on physical examination depend on the severity and stage of the disease. Early on, the examination may be relatively benign with normal range of motion. As the disease progresses, decreased range of motion of the thumb (or other affected joints) can be observed.[2] The grind test (Video 1) can also be helpful in determining the presence of carpometacarpal joint arthritis. It is performed by holding the thumb's metacarpal bone and moving the thumb in a circle while applying gentle axial pressure. Sudden and sharp pain is a positive test. An examiner may also feel crepitus during this maneuver.[2] Grip strength may also be reduced as compared with the contralateral side. The examiner may also find visual deformity with enlargement of the base of the thumb.[1]

Diagnostic Tests

The diagnosis of hand OA can be made based on history and physical examination without imaging. If radiographs are obtained, they are likely to reveal joint space narrowing, osteophyte formation, subchondral sclerosis, and subchondral cyst formation.[1] There is no role for ultrasound or MRI in the standard workup of hand OA unless the presentation is atypical. A history of trauma, prolonged morning stiffness, rapidly worsening symptoms, or obvious inflammation on physical examination may indicate alternative diagnoses and invite further workup, including radiographs.

Treatment

Educating patients is paramount regardless of the severity of disease. This education should include resources describing the nature and course of disease, along with self-management guides.[3] A multidisciplinary approach is important, especially for severe disease. Targeted physical therapy and exercises can help, although it is unclear how much relief this offers compared with other joints affected by OA.[2,3] Splinting can also be considered. Pharmacologic analgesic options include topical nonsteroidal anti-inflammatory drugs (NSAIDs), capsaicin, oral acetaminophen, or oral NSAIDs. Intraarticular injection of corticosteroid is also an option, especially in those who have one or 2 joints that are the cause of their morbidity. Surgery is an option for some patients who have refractory disease.[3]

CLINICAL CARE POINTS

- Hand osteoarthritis is a common cause of pain at the base of the thumb.
- Look for firm nodules at the distal interphalangeal joints and proximal interphalangeal joints as a sign of osteoarthritis.

- Educate patients on self-management and use topical nonsteroidal anti-inflammatory drugs.
- Refer to a hand surgeon if symptoms are severe or refractory.

CARPEL TUNNEL SYNDROME
Background

Carpal tunnel syndrome (CTS) is the most common entrapment neuropathy (nerve damage caused by passage through narrow spaces).[4] The median nerve is compressed when it passes through the carpal tunnel, which is composed of wrist bones, transverse carpal ligament, median nerve, and digital flexor tendons. The overall prevalence is unknown, but some estimate that 10% of the general population will develop CTS at some point in their lives.[4] There is a strong female predominance of the disease, and the risk increases with age.[5] Risk factors for CTS include diabetes, menopause, pregnancy, hypothyroidism, obesity, and repetitive wrist activities, including the use of vibratory tools.[4,5] When evaluating patients with hand numbness as a chief complaint, providers should use the history and physical examination to distinguish the localized nerve entrapment of CTS from a polyneuropathy (from an alternative cause such as vitamin B12 deficiency or diabetes) and a cervical radiculopathy.

Clinical Features

Patients with early CTS report intermittent nocturnal symptoms that include some or all of the following: pain, numbness, tingling, and paresthesia. When the disease progresses, these episodes increase in frequency and begin to occur during the day.[4] Eventually, loss of sensation, muscular weakness, and atrophy occur. The location of the discomfort classically involves the area of the hand that is innervated by the median nerve: palmar aspect of the thumb, index, middle, and the radial half of the fourth finger. In practice, symptoms can vary in location and can include the entire hand, localize to the wrist, or radiate proximally to the forearm, upper arm, and even the shoulder.[4,5] Patients who describe awakening with symptoms followed by shaking their hand to relieve symptoms are describing the flick sign, which is 93% sensitive and 96% specific.[5]

Physical Examination

Before focusing on the hand and wrist, it is important to evaluate for other common causes of neuropathic symptoms, including examination of other peripheral nerves, the entire upper extremity, and the neck. The Spurling test is performed by rotating the head and extending the neck. An axial load is then applied to the head. Eliciting a shocklike sensation suggests a radicular syndrome rather than CTS.[2] This alternative diagnosis may be supported by reduction or absent deep tendon reflexes. In CTS, inspection of the palm may reveal thenar atrophy in severe cases. There are various provocative maneuvers that can be used to evaluate a patient for CTS. Performing more than one increases the accuracy of the evaluation.[5] All of the maneuvers attempt to transiently exacerbate the entrapment and are positive if symptoms are reproduced. Percussion of the carpal tunnel is called Tinel test. Phalen test is forced or passive flexion of the wrist while the elbow is extended for 1 minute. The wrist compression test (Video 2) passively flexes the wrist while direct pressure is applied to the carpal tunnel. It appears that this test has the most sensitivity and specificity.[2]

Diagnosis

The diagnosis of typical CTS can be made clinically without additional testing. When the diagnosis is in question or there is concern for alternative diagnoses, nerve conduction studies may be helpful. Although electrophysiological assessment is relatively sensitive, it can be negative in up to one-third of patients with mild entrapment,[5] even though symptoms may be severe.[4] Ultrasound has been increasingly used for diagnosis as well. This modality can be used to measure the cross-sectional area of the nerve, which has been closely correlated to the severity of disease (a measurement of >9 mm^2 is both sensitive and specific for CTS).[5]

Treatment

Management of CTS depends on the severity of disease. In mild to moderate disease where there has been no impact on muscle strength, conservative/noninvasive measures are reasonable. First, the least invasive and lowest risk intervention is to educate patients about the cause of their disease and counsel them to limit repetitive wrist movements, reduce heavy work activities, and adapt ergonomically friendly habits. Other noninvasive measures include splinting the wrist in order to reduce flexion and extension. This splinting limits the increase in pressure in the carpal tunnel.[2] Initially, splints can be worn full time (as this may improve symptoms more quickly), but this may lead to muscle weakness secondary to disuse and dependence on the splint.[2] Steroid injection is a nonsurgical alternative. This procedure can be done under ultrasound guidance and reduces symptoms and the rate of surgery compared with placebo at 1 year, although most patients in this study still went on to surgery (73% vs 92%).[6] Other nonsurgical alternatives, such as laser therapy and therapeutic ultrasound, are available, although further studies are needed to show efficacy.[4] For severe disease, surgical decompression is recommended. It is helpful to obtain nerve conduction studies before referral for surgical evaluation. Referral to a specialist should take place if a patient has severe CTS with muscle weakness and/or atrophy or if they have persistent symptoms despite conservative management for 6 weeks.

CLINICAL CARE POINTS

- Carpal tunnel syndrome causes neuropathic symptoms of the palm and fingers.
- Perform Tinel, Phalen, and wrist compression tests to try to reproduce symptoms.
- Nerve conduction studies are not needed for typical and mild symptoms.
- Use behavior modification and splinting as first line of treatment.
- Refer to a hand surgeon if there is muscle weakness or atrophy.

GANGLION CYSTS
Background

A common and benign cause of masslike growths of the hand or wrist are ganglion cysts. They usually occur in 20 to 40 year olds with a predominance for women.[7] The cysts are usually located adjacent to tendons or joints, with the dorsal aspect of the wrist (70%) being more common than the volar side of the wrist (20%).[8] The cysts are filled with thick fluid, and there is usually a communication between the cyst and the tendon sheath or joint through a stalk.[9] Historically, they were called bible cysts because of the old wives' tale suggesting that they could be eliminated by a direct blow with a bible (causing rupture).

Clinical Features

Most patients bring a ganglion cyst to the attention of their physician after it has been present for months or years. They are typically asymptomatic,[9] although occasionally they can cause discomfort depending on the location and size.[2] The size of the cyst typically fluctuates and may be related to activity. It is unusual for a cyst to continue to increase in size.

Physical Examination

It is not unusual for a patient to report a mass that is not obvious to the examiner at the time of the visit because of fluctuations in size. It may become more prominent with wrist flexion or extension. When present, the cyst is usually uniform, smooth, firm, non-tender, and translucent to light. It is also minimally mobile.[9]

Diagnosis

The diagnosis of a ganglion cyst is made clinically. Radiographs are only needed if underlying bony pathologic condition is suspected. Imaging, such as MRI or ultrasound, should be reserved for patients with an unusual history (continuous growth, preceding trauma, or constant pain) or atypical examination (unusual location, multilobular masses).

Treatment

The previous practice of direct trauma to induce rupture is no longer in favor.[9] Because most cysts are asymptomatic, reassurance is usually sufficient for many patients. There is a relatively high rate of spontaneous resolution (40%–58%) within 6 years of diagnosis.[8] Thus, if discomfort is present, conservative management with immobilization and oral analgesia may offer relief until the cyst decreases in size or resolves. For symptoms that persist, aspiration alone or aspiration with corticosteroid injection can offer relief, although there are high rates of recurrence.[8] Of note, because the fluid is usually quite viscous, a large-bore needle is recommended. Surgical excision in the hands of an experienced surgeon is an additional option for patients with persistent symptoms. This approach leads to a low rate of recurrence.[8,9]

CLINICAL CARE POINTS

- Ganglion cysts are usually asymptomatic masses that fluctuate in size and are found on the dorsal aspect of the wrist.
- No imaging is necessary for diagnosis unless the cyst continuously grows or is multilobular.
- Reassurance is first-line therapy; many cysts spontaneously resolve.

PLANTAR FASCIITIS
Background

Plantar fasciitis is the most common cause of heel pain with 10% of the general population experiencing this problem in their lifetime.[10] Risk factors include body mass index more than 27, running, or prolonged standing. It is considered to be an overuse injury that leads to degenerative changes, including microtears in the contracted fascia.[10,11] Thus, the name is a misnomer because there is a paucity of inflammation.

Clinical Features

Patients typically complain of anteromedial heel pain. It is characterized as sharp and usually is at its worst upon initiation of ambulation after a period of rest (such as upon wakening in the morning or after prolonged sitting). The pain gradually improves with activity.[10] Historically, changes in a patient's ambulation routine, such as starting a new exercise regimen or wearing new footwear, may precede onset. It is unusual to have numbness or paresthesia with plantar fasciitis.

Physical Examination

On physical examination, patients are tender to palpation on the medial side of the calcaneus. They may also be tender with forced dorsiflexion of the toes at the metatarsophalangeal joints while the ankle is stabilized: the windlass test.[10] This maneuver is insensitive but specific. The physical examination should be performed with a goal of seeking an alternative diagnosis, such as a calcaneal stress fracture. Squeezing the posterior one-third of the calcaneus between the thumb and index finger (calcaneal squeeze test)[12] should not reproduce pain and can help rule out a calcaneal stress fracture.[13]

Diagnosis

Plantar fasciitis is a clinical diagnosis. Imaging is reserved for patients who do not improve or who have atypical history or examination findings that indicate possible underlying bony pathologic condition, such as stress fracture.

Treatment

It is important to emphasize to patients that there is no quick fix. Treatment is usually prolonged; it may take months for symptoms to resolve.[13] The vast majority (80%) of patients have resolution of symptoms with conservative treatment (over-the-counter analgesics and exercises).[11] Identifying and modifying behavior that may have contributed to the condition is important. Patients should be encouraged to avoid being barefoot, even using folded washcloths to support their arches in the shower. Basic stretching can be accomplished at home, including just rolling a tennis ball under the arch of the foot, and are described well by Becker and Childress.[11] Adding orthotics to provide improved heel padding or arch support is also effective.

For patients who fail to improve, the benefit for more invasive interventions is unclear. A Cochrane review found that corticosteroid injection may provide minimal relief for 1 month, but no difference long term.[14] Platelet-rich plasma (PRP) injection has been proposed as a treatment for multiple degenerative conditions. A recent review of 15 studies that compared PRP and corticosteroid injection showed that PRP was more effective in reducing pain when evaluated at 6 months and 12 months. In the short term, there was no difference between the 2 groups.[15]

Patients should be referred to a foot and ankle specialist if symptoms severely impact daily activities or if they are recalcitrant to conservative treatments after a few months. Imaging or further workup should be initiated if there are neurologic signs or symptoms, such as numbness or paresthesia, or if bony pathologic condition, such as a calcaneal stress fracture, is suspected.

CLINICAL CARE POINTS

- Plantar fasciitis is a common cause of heel pain that is worse after prolonged rest and improves with ambulation.
- Use the calcaneal squeeze test to evaluate for stress fracture.
- Basic stretching and heel support resolve most cases.
- Refer to foot specialist if symptoms do not improve after several months.

ONYCHOMYCOSIS
Background

Onychomycosis is a common disorder of toenails that has an estimated prevalence of 6% to 14% in the general population, with an increased prevalence in warm and humid climates.[11] It is caused by an infection of the toenail by dermatophytes, nondermatophyte molds, or yeasts.[16] There is an increased prevalence of onychomycosis with advanced age, family history of the same, immunosuppression, diabetes, peripheral vascular disease, tinea pedis, and smoking.[16] Wearing occlusive footwear also contributes to the development of the condition.

Clinical Features

Patients with onychomycosis have toenails that are discolored (yellow, white, or brown), thick, brittle, and separated from the nail bed (onycholysis).[16] Usually, the infection is limited and is mostly a cosmetic condition, but occasionally, onychomycosis can cause pain and even impact a patient's ability to ambulate. Most frequently, patients experience social embarrassment that accompanies the appearance of the abnormal toenails.

Diagnosis

Toenails with the changes described above raise clinical suspicion for onychomycosis. Most experts recommend confirming the diagnosis with bedside testing with potassium hydroxide (KOH) preparation microscopy of nail clipping followed by fungal culture. Other techniques, such as histopathology, polymerase chain reaction, and flow cytometry, are also available.[16] Confirming the diagnosis may help tailor treatment and evaluate for alternative diagnosis, such as nail psoriasis, trauma, and lichen planus. Unfortunately, onychomycosis and these other disorders may coexist, and positive testing for infection does not exclude an alternative diagnosis.

Treatment

Toenails grow at approximately 1 to 2 mm per month.[17] Therefore, it is important to counsel patients that treatment of onychomycosis takes time. Several treatments are available for the treatment of onychomycosis. Opinions regarding who should be treated vary widely. Over-the-counter topical solutions are ineffective. Prescription topical medications have significantly lower cure rates than systemic oral antifungal agents. Even the systemic agents have a recurrence rate of 20% to 25%.[17] Lipner and Scher[17] suggest treating onychomycosis with systemic medications if more than 4 nails are affected, if there is proximal subungual involvement, or if there are factors that propend poor prognosis, such as immunosuppression. Both terbinafine and itraconazole have Food and Drug Administration approval for the treatment of onychomycosis. Terbinafine is usually favored because of higher cure rates and fewer drug interactions.[17] It is the author's opinion that if there is minimal impact to the patient, reassurance and monitoring is an acceptable approach.

If there is pain associated with onychomycosis, a patient can be referred to a specialist (podiatry or dermatology) with the purpose of removing the thickened and painful part of the nail. Furthermore, negative diagnostic testing should be referred to a specialist in order to help elucidate the cause of the nail changes.

CLINICAL CARE POINTS

- Onychomycosis is a condition that is mostly cosmetic but can cause pain and social embarrassment.
- Nail clippings can be evaluated with KOH and microscopy and be sent for fungal culture.
- Over-the-counter remedies are ineffective. Both topical and systemic treatments have high recurrence rates.

MORTON INTERDIGITAL NEUROMA
Background

A common cause of plantar foot pain, an interdigital neuroma is a bulge in the interdigital nerve proximal to the bifurcation into the digital nerves that results in a syndrome that is described in later discussion.[18] Is it not completely known what causes the formation of the neuroma, but several theories exist, including chronic traction damage, chronic inflammation from bursitis, chronic compression, and ischemia.[19] Interdigital neuromas are much more common in women than men and usually present in middle-aged individuals.[18] The neuroma is found to be bilateral in one-fifth of patients. The most common location is in the third interdigital space (between the third and fourth distal metatarsals) in two-thirds of patients, followed by the second space. It is rare for a neuroma to be present in multiple interdigital spaces.[18]

Clinical Features

Patients with Morton neuroma complain of burning, sharp, or shocklike pain on the plantar surface of the foot between metatarsal heads. This pain can radiate distally to the 2 adjacent toes or proximally.[18] The pain worsens with tight-fitting footwear or high heels. Patients sometimes also complain of numbness in the same area.

Physical Examination

Direct palpation of the involved interdigital space may reproduce the reported pain. A painful clicking sensation may also be found by palpating the interdigital space while simultaneously squeezing the metatarsal joints (Mulder sign). This maneuver has been shown to be 61% to 98% sensitive.[20,21] It is essential to confirm that palpation of the metatarsal head is not tender. This finding would be inconsistent with a Morton neuroma and should lead to further evaluation.

Diagnosis

A history and physical examination that are consistent with the diagnosis of an interdigital neuroma are sufficient for diagnosis. Di Caprio and colleagues[18] suggest injection of a local anesthetic if Mulder sign is negative to confirm the diagnosis.[18] If that does not relieve pain, alternative diagnoses should be entertained. Imaging is usually unhelpful in the diagnosis and management. Specifically, MRI is neither sensitive nor specific. For patients with atypical features, such as more than 1 web space involvement, ultrasound is the imaging modality of choice. Ultrasound findings include greater fascia thickness and reduced echogenicity.[10]

Treatment

It is reasonable to take an escalating management approach to treating interdigital neuromas. Conservative treatment, such as using plantar orthosis, for metatarsal offloading, and wearing wider footwear lead to improvement of symptoms

Table 1
Summary of the 6 common symptoms involving the hands and feet

Diagnosis	Most Common Location of Pain	Typical Examination	Diagnosis	Primary Care Treatment	Refer to Specialist
Hand osteoarthritis	Base of thumb	Heberden and Bouchard nodes, positive grind test	Clinical, radiographs show joint space narrowing and osteophytes	Behavioral modification, exercises, topical NSAIDs	Conservative management fails
Carpal tunnel syndrome	Palm, first 3 digits. Flick sign	Positive Phalen, Tinel, wrist compression tests, thenar atrophy if severe	Clinical, nerve conduction studies if severe	Behavioral modification, splinting	Muscle weakness or atrophy, failure of conservative management after 6 wk
Ganglion cyst	None	Spherical, uniform, smooth, translucent mass on dorsal wrist	Clinical	Reassurance, immobilization, aspiration ± steroid injection	Continuous growth, pain that does not improve with conservative management
Plantar fasciitis	Anteromedial heel	+ Windlass test, negative calcaneal squeeze	Clinical	Home exercises, OTC analgesia, orthotics	Severe symptoms, failure to respond after 3–6 mo of conservative management
Onychomycosis	None	Yellow, thick, brittle nails	Clinical ± KOH microscopy and fungal culture	None, prescription topical or systemic antifungal therapy	Pain, negative diagnostic workup
Morton neuroma	Between third and fourth distal metatarsal	+ Mulder sign	Clinical ± ultrasound	Orthotic for metatarsal offloading	Failure to improve, pain at metatarsal head

See text for description of examination maneuvers.
Abbreviation: OTC, over the counter.

in 32% of patients.[22] Corticosteroid injection relieves symptoms in a third of patients. Most of these patients achieve resolution of symptoms without recurrence.[18] Botulinum toxin A injection appears to be more effective than corticosteroid injection. Alcohol injections have an even higher rate of initial response, but a concomitant increase in relapse.[18] For those who failed to improve with nonsurgical approaches, surgical resection of the neuroma showed an approximately 90% success rate.[19] If patients do not respond to the conservative management outlined above, referral to a specialist for more invasive interventions is suggested.

CLINICAL CARE POINTS

- Neuropathic pain in the interdigital area between metatarsal heads is consistent with a neuroma.
- Mulder sign (palpating the interdigital space while simultaneously squeezing the metatarsal joints) is a sensitive and specific examination finding.
- Imaging is not required for diagnosis.
- Resection of the neuroma is highly effective if nonsurgical interventions fail.

SUMMARY

Table 1 summarizes the details of these 6 common symptoms involving the hands and feet. The complaints are common in primary care. The diagnoses of all of these conditions can be made using the patient history and a targeted physical examination. Rarely are more advanced imaging or diagnostic techniques necessary. Furthermore, conservative, nonsurgical treatments are usually the first step in management.

DISCLOSURE

The authors have nothing to disclose.

SUPPLEMENTARY DATA

Supplementary data to this article can be found online at https://doi.org/10.1016/j.mcna.2020.08.016.

REFERENCES

1. Marshall M, Watt FE, Vincent TL, et al. Hand osteoarthritis: clinical phenotypes, molecular mechanisms and disease management. Nat Rev Rheumatol 2018; 14(11):641–56.

2. Darowish M, Sharma J. Evaluation and treatment of chronic hand conditions. Med Clin North Am 2014;98(4):801–15, xii.

3. Kloppenburg M, Kroon FP, Blanco FJ, et al. 2018 update of the EULAR recommendations for the management of hand osteoarthritis. Ann Rheum Dis 2019; 78(1):16–24.

4. Padua L, Coraci D, Erra C, et al. Carpal tunnel syndrome: clinical features, diagnosis, and management. Lancet Neurol 2016;15(12):1273–84.

5. Wipperman J, Goerl K. Carpal tunnel syndrome: diagnosis and management. Am Fam Physician 2016;94(12):993–9.

6. Atroshi I, Flondell M, Hofer M, et al. Methylprednisolone injections for the carpal tunnel syndrome: a randomized, placebo-controlled trial. Ann Intern Med 2013; 159(5):309–17.

7. Gregush RE, Habusta SF. Ganglion cyst. In: StatPearls. Treasure Island (FL): Stat-Pearls Publishing; 2020.

8. Suen M, Fung B, Lung CP. Treatment of ganglion cysts. ISRN Orthop 2013;2013: 940615.

9. Nahra ME, Bucchieri JS. Ganglion cysts and other tumor related conditions of the hand and wrist. Hand Clin 2004;20(3):249–60, v.

10. Trojian T, Tucker AK. Plantar fasciitis. Am Fam Physician 2019;99(12):744–50.

11. Becker BA, Childress MA. Common foot problems: over-the-counter treatments and home care. Am Fam Physician 2018;98(5):298–303.

12. Weber JM, Vidt LG, Gehl RS, et al. Calcaneal stress fractures. Clin Podiatr Med Surg 2005;22(1):45–54.

13. Albano AW, Nelson V. Approaching foot and ankle injuries in the ambulatory setting. Prim Care 2020;47(1):133–45.

14. David JA, Sankarapandian V, Christopher PR, et al. Injected corticosteroids for treating plantar heel pain in adults. Cochrane Database Syst Rev 2017;6: CD009348.

15. Alkhatib N, Salameh M, Ahmed AF, et al. Platelet-rich plasma versus corticoste-roids in the treatment of chronic plantar fasciitis: a systematic review and meta-analysis of prospective comparative studies. J Foot Ankle Surg 2020;59(3): 546–52.

16. Gupta AK, Stec N, Summerbell RC, et al. Onychomycosis: a review. J Eur Acad Dermatol Venereol 2020. https://doi.org/10.1111/jdv.16394.

17. Lipner SR, Scher RK. Onychomycosis: treatment and prevention of recurrence. J Am Acad Dermatol 2019;80(4):853–67.

18. Di Caprio F, Meringolo R, Shehab Eddine M, et al. Morton's interdigital neuroma of the foot: a literature review. Foot Ankle Surg 2018;24(2):92–8.

19. Valisena S, Petri GJ, Ferrero A. Treatment of Morton's neuroma: a systematic re-view. Foot Ankle Surg 2017. https://doi.org/10.1016/j.fas.2017.03.010.

20. Mahadevan D, Venkatesan M, Bhatt R, et al. Diagnostic accuracy of clinical tests for Morton's neuroma compared with ultrasonography. J Foot Ankle Surg 2015; 54(4):549–53.

21. Pastides P, El-Sallakh S, Charalambides C. Morton's neuroma: a clinical versus radiological diagnosis. Foot Ankle Surg 2012;18(1):22–4.

22. Matthews BG, Hurn SE, Harding MP, et al. The effectiveness of non-surgical inter-ventions for common plantar digital compressive neuropathy (Morton's neuroma): a systematic review and meta-analysis. J Foot Ankle Res 2019;12:12.

A Symptom-Directed Paradigm for the Evaluation and Management of Upper Respiratory Tract Infections

Fred N. Pelzman, MD*, Judy Tung, MD

KEYWORDS

- Upper respiratory tract infections • Common cold • Bronchitis • Sinusitis
- Pharyngitis • Otitis • Evaluation and management • Symptoms

KEY POINTS

- Upper respiratory tract infections account for significant burdens on the health care system and individual patients.
- Effective evaluation involves using primarily history to assess the primary sites of involvement, with physical examination offering supportive data and helping to confirm or refute presumptive diagnoses.
- Laboratory testing, imaging, and subspecialty involvement are rarely necessary, but can be useful in specific syndromes and conditions.
- Certain mimics of upper respiratory tract infection symptoms should be considered, and for each one, there are important diagnoses and emergent conditions that are critical to consider.
- Treatment should address patient preferences, symptom-directed care, counseling about avoiding overprescribing, and close follow-up.

INTRODUCTION

Upper respiratory tract infections (URTIs) rank with hypertension, diabetes, asthma, and low back pain as the bread and butter of the outpatient practitioner. Symptoms localized to the upper respiratory tract, including those of infectious and noninfectious causes, are perennially in the top 10 list of reasons that adult patients seek medical guidance.[1] URTI symptoms account for significant morbidity and health care resource

Division of General Internal Medicine, Department of Medicine, Weill Cornell Medicine, 505 East 70th Street, New York, NY 10021, USA
* Corresponding author.
E-mail address: fpelzman@med.cornell.edu
Twitter: @Dr_Pelzman (F.N.P.); @JudyTungMD (J.T.)

Med Clin N Am 105 (2021) 199–212
https://doi.org/10.1016/j.mcna.2020.08.020
0025-7125/21/© 2020 Elsevier Inc. All rights reserved.

utilization. The associated health care costs, as well as societal costs owing to time missed at work and school and decreased productivity, are enormous as well.[2,3]

The upper respiratory tract entails everything above the lower respiratory tract: the nose, sinuses, ears, oropharynx, tonsils, larynx, epiglottis, trachea, and upper bronchi. When these areas become inflamed or infected, they result in rhinitis, sinusitis, otitis, pharyngitis, tonsillitis, laryngitis, epiglottitis, tracheitis, and bronchitis. Most respiratory infections are caused by a large group of viruses (adenovirus, coronavirus, rhinovirus, human metapneumovirus, enterovirus, influenza, parainfluenza, respiratory syncytial virus), although certain bacteria and other (rare) pathogens can cause URTIs and should not be missed. Bacterial infections can be primary or secondary when they occur after protective defensive mechanisms have been battered and denuded by a virus, leaving anatomic tissues open to a bacterial assault.

Distinguishing viral, bacterial, and other causes can be challenging but is critical to achieving optimal patient outcomes. Thankfully, most URTI are self-limited and respond to symptom-directed care along with close monitoring.

The appearance of COVID-19, caused by the novel coronavirus severe acute respiratory syndrome coronavirus 2, has likely permanently altered how patients with upper respiratory tract symptoms are evaluated and managed. In the midst of the current pandemic, in areas where the disease is highly prevalent and where communities have yet to achieve herd immunity, infection with this virus must be considered in every patient presenting with URTI symptoms. Initial experience has informed us that COVID-19 patients present with high and persistent fevers, cough and shortness of breath, severe malaise and myalgias, loss of sense of taste and smell, and diarrhea.[4] However, much is still unknown about this disease, and because information is rapidly evolving, the specifics of the evaluation and management of COVID-19 are not included in this article.

INITIAL EVALUATION

Evaluating patients with upper respiratory tract symptoms is best done in a systematic manner. Patients can present with a broad range of symptoms, including runny nose, nasal congestion, itchy eyes and nose, red eyes, ear pain, muffled or decreased hearing, vertigo, sore throat, difficulty swallowing, sinus pain, tooth pain, cough, sputum production, fever, fatigue, shortness of breath, wheezing, hoarse voice, myalgias, and malaise. The history of present illness should, however, reveal which symptoms predominate. Asking which symptoms bother the patient the most can provide the necessary clues to the clinical diagnosis (**Table 1**). Further testing, including disease-specific laboratory tests and imaging, as well as consultations with subspecialists, is seldom warranted.

Additional elements of the history should include queries into underlying medical conditions, such as asthma, chronic obstructive pulmonary disease, diabetes, heart failure, and other cardiac issues, as these may put patients at increased risk for decompensation, and the conditions themselves may flare up. Patients should also be evaluated for immunocompromising states from conditions such as HIV/AIDS and cancer, or from immune modulating drugs, such as chemotherapy and corticosteroids. The elderly may present with widely variable symptoms and may simply show changes in behavior, have decreased levels of alertness, or loss of appetite.

Extrinsic factors that should be explored include recent travel history, exposure to ill contacts, occupation (such as working in a preschool), and immunization status. Information on smoking and alcohol use should also be collected. Awareness of any illnesses currently prevalent in the community can also be highly informative.

Table 1
Differential diagnosis by symptom predominance

	Common Cold	Influenza	COVID-19	Strep Throat	Mononucleosis	Otitis Media	Viral Sinusitis	Bacterial Sinusitis	Bronchitis	Pneumonia	Allergic Rhinitis	GERD
Fever	+	+++	+++	+++	+++	+	++	++	+	+++		
Headache	+	+	+	+	+	+	++	+++	+		+	
Myalgia	+	+++	+++	+	++	+	+	+	+	++	+	
Malaise	+	+++	+++	+	+++	+	+	+	+	++	+	
Rhinorrhea	++	++	+			+	++	++	+		++	
Congestion	++	++	+			+++	+++	+++	+		++	
Anosmia	+		+++				++	++			+	
Ear pain	+					+++	++	++				
Hearing loss	+					+++	+	+				
Sore throat	+	++	+++	+++	+++	+	+	+	+		+	++
Facial or tooth pain							++	+++				
Cough	++	++	+++				+	+	+++	+++	++	++
Wheeze	+	++							++	++	++	+

(+), minor; (++), intermediate; (+++), major.

Finally, patients should be queried about what treatments and medications they have already tried to date, how effective these were, and whether things are improving or are getting worse. It is also important to explore the prior course of similar illnesses. If symptoms have persisted beyond 3 weeks, the evaluation should likely shift to consideration of other causes, such as noninfectious, subacute, or chronic syndromes.

The physical examination in patients presenting with upper respiratory symptoms should start with a general impression of how they look, including evidence of dehydration in the form of dry mucous membrane or loss of skin turgor, as this can give insight into how well a patient is tolerating the symptoms of an underlying infection. Vital signs should include oxygen saturation and peak flow if patients have asthma or experience wheezing, in addition to blood pressure, pulse, temperature, and respiratory rate. The HEENT examination should look for sinus tenderness, purulent discharge in the nares, bulging or ruptured tympanic membranes, stridor, and enlarged or tender adenopathy. A lung examination should always be done to exclude lower respiratory tract infection or a significant exacerbation of asthma. At this time, auscultation, percussion, egophony, and even the search for tactile fremitus can be useful. Additional attention should be given to the skin for rashes and the abdomen for splenomegaly especially if the differential diagnosis includes Epstein-Barr virus (EBV)/infectious mononucleosis. Signs of other severe imitators, such as meningitis, photophobia, stiff neck, or disproportionally severe headaches, should also be elicited.

SPECIFIC UPPER RESPIRATORY TRACT INFECTIONS SYNDROMES

The above approach usually narrows the evaluation down to specific conditions or syndromes, which are reviewed in the following section. Again, the dominant URTI symptoms can help guide the astute clinician to the most precise diagnosis and treatment.

EAR PAIN: OTITIS

Patients with almost any type of URTI can present with ear pain, raising the possibility of acute otitis media. Inflammation along the eustachian tube leads to the buildup of pressure that manifests as ear pain, decreased or muffled hearing, or vertigo. Although otitis in children is often viral and resolves without treatment, in adults, especially those with a history of recurrent ear infections or anatomic abnormalities, bacterial causes should be considered. Otoscopic examination should include a search for diffuse redness, bulge or rupture of tympanic membranes, loss of the tympanic light reflex, and severe inflammation in the external auditory canal. Checking for reduced mobility of the tympanic membrane with pneumatoscopy is rarely done in adults. Ensuring no deep-seated local infections are present, such as mastoiditis (with local bony tenderness) or meningitis (with stiff neck or photophobia), is also important. Laboratory testing or imaging is rarely indicated. Referral to otorhinolaryngologists is necessary only in chronic or severe cases, or when there is hearing loss or tympanic membrane rupture. Important alternative diagnoses beyond infections include temporomandibular joint disorders, traumatic or idiopathic tympanic membrane rupture, otitis externa, and foreign bodies in the external auditory canal.[5]

SINUS PAIN AND HEADACHE: RHINITIS, SINUSITIS

Patients presenting with symptoms that predominantly involve the nasal sinuses will often have headaches, sinus pressure, sinus pain, anosmia, ageusia, rhinorrhea, purulent nasal discharge, and upper tooth pain. Patients may report multiple sinus infections in the past or a history of nasal septal deviation. As with most URTIs, infections of the sinuses are almost always primarily viral in origin. However, a phenomenon known as "double sickening" can occur: an initial illness that is followed by clinical improvement, and then followed by a worsening of symptoms may represent bacterial "superinfection."[6] Fever greater than 39°C, prolonged duration of symptoms, for example, greater than 10 days, and facial or tooth pain lasting greater than 3 days are concerning signs for bacterial superinfection.[7] Useful findings on physical examination include purulent discharge in the nares, focal tenderness to either percussion or deep digital pressure across the maxillary, ethmoid, or frontal sinuses. Transillumination of the nasal sinuses, cultures of nasal or sinus discharge, radiographs, or computed tomographic scans rarely add additional information. Referrals to an ear, nose, and throat (ENT) physician for direct examination with nasal endoscopy should be reserved for severe, refractory, or recurrent disease, or where underlying pathologic condition is thought to be contributing (ie, deviated nasal septum, nasal polyps, other structural abnormalities).[8] Rapidly progressing symptoms involving eye pain or visual changes may suggest deeper tissue penetration and should invoke consideration of invasive bacterial or fungal sinusitis (eg, *Naegleria fowleri*, the "brain-eating ameba"). Immunocompromising conditions, including diabetes, HIV/AIDS, and certain malignant conditions, such as myeloproliferative disorders, may also put patients at increased risk of invasive sinus disease. In rare cases, bacterial sinusitis can even progress to meningitis.

SORE THROAT: PHARYNGITIS, TONSILLITIS, LARYNGITIS, EPIGLOTTITIS

Sore throat is often the first symptom to appear in the common cold, swiftly followed by runny nose, sneezing, itchy red eyes, nasal congestion, and hoarseness. The patient may describe throat pain as a burning sensation at rest or when swallowing. Examination should include inspection of the oropharynx for ulcers and tonsillar exudate and palpation of the neck for adenopathy. High fevers that accompany sore throat are more often associated with influenza or strep throat. Diagnosing strep throat, caused by group A β-hemolytic *Streptococcus pyogenes* (GABHS), is one of the main diagnostic challenges but one for which there is well-established evidence.[9–12] When strep throat is prevalent in the community, the use of the clinical decision rule known as the modified Centor criteria can help guide the clinician to a diagnosis (**Box 1**). This tool is useful in deciding who to treat, and who needs additional testing with point-of-care rapid antigen testing for GABHS or with a throat culture. Empiric antibiotics can be given when clinical suspicion is high enough (4 or greater on modified Centor score) without further testing, as long as other causes that mimic these same criteria have been clinically ruled out (acute HIV infection, gonococcal pharyngitis, mononucleosis). Although the sensitivity of the modified Centor criteria may not fully support this pathway, it is often seen in clinical practice.[13] Other bacterial causes of pharyngitis (such as group C and group G *Streptococcus* or *Arcanobacterium haemolyticum*) can cause similar symptoms but rarely suppurative complications. Most importantly, they do not cause the systemic complications of strep throat, such as rheumatic fever or glomerulonephritis.

There are several other infectious diseases that particularly affect the throat and should always be considered in the differential diagnosis.[14] Mononucleosis, caused by EBV, presents with fevers, sore throat, significantly enlarged tonsils, swollen glands, and often a maculopapular rash. Patients may have an enlarged spleen on examination as well as petechiae on the palate. Complete blood count (CBC) can reveal

---

Box 1
Centor criteria for the diagnosis of strep throat owing to group A β-hemolytic *Streptococcus pyogenes*

Patients are judged on 4 criteria, with 1 point added for each positive criterion[9]:
    Absence of cough: 1 point
    Tonsillar exudates: 1 point
    History of fever or current fever: 1 point
    Enlarged tender anterior cervical lymph nodes: 1 point

The modified Centor criteria also incorporate the patient's age[10,11]:
    Age less than 15: add 1 point
    Age greater than 44: subtract 1 point

Scoring: Scores range from −1 to 5

Guidelines for management based on score:
- −1, 0, or 1 point: No antibiotic or throat culture necessary (risk of GABHS infection <10%)
- 2 or 3 points: Perform throat culture and treat with an appropriate antibiotic if culture is positive (risk of GABHS infection 32% if 3 points, 15% if 2 points)
- 4 or 5 points: Consider rapid strep testing and/or throat culture (risk of GABHS infection ∼56%)

Data from Refs.[9–11]

---

atypical lymphocytes and a heterophile antibody test (Monospot), or an EBV antibody panel can help. The acute HIV seroconversion reaction, gonococcal pharyngitis, and acute herpes simplex infection of the pharynx should also be considered, and patients should be asked about a history of unprotected receptive oral sex.

Epiglottitis is primarily a bacterial infection in children, but in adults, it can be viral or bacterial. In addition to a sore throat, patients will present with fevers, "muffled" or hoarse voice, and drooling. The latter, along with stridor or any other signs of impending airway compromise, should prompt emergency evaluation in a setting with the capacity for airway management.[15,16]

Deep tissue infections of the throat and neck can mimic more common causes of pharyngitis; severe symptoms, abnormal swelling of local tissues, trismus, or other signs of systemic illness should raise these concerns. Other dangerous causes to consider are the suppurative complications of strep throat (including peritonsillar, retropharyngeal, pharyngeal, and submandibular abscesses), and rarely, diphtheria.

Mimics of infectious causes include gastroesophageal reflux disease (GERD) and laryngopharyngeal reflux (LPR), thyroiditis, postnasal drip, and lodged foreign body or abrasions (such as from a swallowed fish bone).

COUGH: BRONCHITIS, TRACHEITIS, PNEUMONIA

In evaluating patients with primarily cough symptoms, the clinician must distinguish minor viral conditions, such as the common cold and bronchitis, from more severe infections, such as influenza, pertussis, COVID-19, and bacterial pneumonia.[17] Fever, wheezing, tachypnea, and shortness of breath could be signs of more serious causes.[18] Patients with asthma may experience exacerbation of their disease, but even those without asthma may develop transient reactive airway disease in the setting of these infections.

Sputum can be described by patients as clear, purulent, blood-tinged, and with a wide range of shades, consistencies, and colors; very little about these characteristics offer useful information that can lead to specific diagnoses,[19] although the classic sputum characteristics of *Streptococcus pneumoniae* ("rust-colored") or *Klebsiella pneumoniae* ("red currant jelly") should prompt consideration of a chest radiograph. Frank purulence or a new change in sputum may also make one consider secondary bacterial superinfection of a previously viral bronchitis.

Influenza is an important consideration in patients presenting with cough during cold and flu season and presents as high fevers and severe muscle aches in addition to sore throat, congestion, and fatigue. Patients often are able to relate the exact hour their symptoms began and describe being "hit by a truck." Point-of-care rapid flu tests to detect influenza A and influenza B, which have great sensitivities and specificities,[20] can be useful to confirm a diagnosis when necessary, although treatment decisions are usually made clinically. Respiratory pathogen panels obtained by nasal or oropharyngeal swabs can be sent to detect numerous viruses and some bacteria, but these are more useful in the inpatient setting to cohort patients or when the clinical team needs to know with certainty which virus it is.

Other laboratory testing that is potentially useful for the evaluation of lower respiratory tract infections, such as bacterial pneumonia, include a CBC and procalcitonin, an inflammatory marker that is induced by certain bacterial toxins, including *S pneumoniae* and *Haemophilus influenzae*. Algorithms that include the use of procalcitonin have been proven to eliminate unnecessary or prolonged antibiotic courses, although its utility has not been fully realized in the outpatient setting.[21]

Imaging in patients presenting with cough should be reserved for suspicion of pulmonary pathologic condition. Subspecialty consultation by ENT or Pulmonary should be considered for refractory cases of cough, or when an emergency/life-threatening diagnosis is a likely possibility.

Finally, many other conditions can produce cough, and these include GERD/LPR, postnasal drip/allergies, vocal cord polyps and other lesions, use of ACE inhibitors, aspiration, bronchiolitis, cough variant asthma, pulmonary embolism, heart failure, tuberculosis, lung cancer, or other pulmonary diseases.

"DON'T MISS" DIAGNOSES

There are several infectious causes for which an accurate diagnosis significantly changes management and patient outcomes.

Rapid diagnosis of influenza enables the use of influenza-specific antiviral therapy. Even if the window of treatment opportunity has passed, closer monitoring is crucial, given its higher morbidity and mortality. Similarly, an accurate diagnosis of pneumonia leads to appropriate antibiotic therapy.[22] The constellation of symptoms associated with an acute HIV seroconversion reaction can mimic an influenza-like illness; this includes fever, myalgias, sore throat, diffuse rash, headaches, and often widespread adenopathy. Early diagnosis of acute HIV has great implications for the patient and is an important public health intervention.

Cough with paroxysms of "barking" and posttussive emesis should prompt consideration for pertussis, or whooping cough. Treatment with an appropriate antibiotic may shorten the postinfectious cough that many patients suffer from for prolonged periods of time (the "cough of 100 days"). Throat culture has poor and variable sensitivity; polymerase chain reaction testing may be more appropriate to send.[23] Many comprehensive respiratory panels either explicitly test for pertussis or do so in the background and report out if positive.

MANAGEMENT OF UPPER RESPIRATORY TRACT INFECTIONS

Unfortunately, there is often a sense of frustration between patients and providers over the management and treatment of URTIs. Patients want their suffering to be taken seriously, and providers feel pressured to prescribe medications, such as antibiotics or opioids. In the following section, the authors review the evidence for antibiotics and other commonly used therapies.

ANTIBIOTICS

Because the common cold is the most frequent cause of upper respiratory infections and because colds are viral in nature, there is intuitively little to no role for antibiotics. This finding is in fact corroborated by evidence from multiple trials demonstrating no benefit from antibiotics for colds even when the nasal discharge or sputum is purulent.[24] For specific URTIs, including bronchitis, pharyngitis, otitis, and sinusitis, the data for antibiotics are a bit more complex.

Acute *bronchitis* is one of the most common diagnoses encountered, estimated at 10% of all ambulatory visits.[7] Although most pathogens implicated in acute bronchitis are viral, certain bacteria, such as *Mycoplasma pneumoniae*, *Chlamydia pneumoniae*, and *Bordetella pertussis*, are sometimes causative. Because signs and symptoms cannot reliably distinguish bacterial from viral bronchitis, empiric antibiotics are tempting. In fact, 71% of visits for acute bronchitis result in a prescription for antibiotics.[25] Unfortunately, trials have demonstrated limited benefit for this practice. A systematic review of 17 randomized controlled trials involving more than 5000 patients showed no difference in antibiotics over placebo. At best, there appears to be a reduction in cough duration by half a day (over an 8- to 10-day period).[26] This modest benefit in the face of the greater potential for harm has the American College of Physicians and the Centers for Disease Control and Prevention (CDC) advising against antibiotics for patients with acute uncomplicated bronchitis.[7]

Although most acute *pharyngitis* is also viral in origin, here there are distinguishing signs and symptoms that allow clinicians to predict the likelihood of bacterial causes, specifically group A *Streptococcus*. The Centor criteria teach that oropharyngeal exudate and absence of cough in the setting of fever and adenopathy predict strep throat. For confirmed group A streptococcal pharyngitis, the Infectious Disease Society of America recommends an appropriate narrow-spectrum antibiotic, such as penicillin or amoxicillin (or for those with penicillin allergies, a first-generation cephalosporin or clindamycin) usually for 10 days.[27] This antibiotic course can shorten the duration of symptoms by up to 2 days, but more importantly, may prevent complications, such as acute rheumatic fever and peritonsillar abscess.

Acute *otitis media* occurs more commonly in children than in adults, and the strategy differs between these 2 populations. In children, because a quarter of cases are attributable to viral pathogens and because in many children's symptoms resolve without treatment, initial observation is recommended by the American Academy of Pediatrics and the American Academy of Family Physicians. In adults, because complication rates from otitis media are higher, antibiotics that cover *S pneumoniae*, *H influenza*, and *Staphylococcus aureus*, such as amoxicillin/clavulanate, are more often considered. Topical antibiotics (usually also containing an anti-inflammatory agent) are adequate for otitis externa, inflammation, and infection limited to the external ear canal.

Acute *rhinosinusitis* nearly always begins as a viral infection. Bacterial rhinosinusitis is a secondary infection resulting from obstruction of the sinuses, impaired mucosal clearance, and resultant bacterial overgrowth. Although less than 2% of viral sinusitis is complicated by bacterial sinusitis, 80% of ambulatory visits for sinusitis results in a prescription for antibiotics.[28] A systematic review of 15 trials involving more than 3000 participants demonstrated that nearly half of patients recover from their illness in

1 week and two-thirds recover in 2 weeks without antibiotics. Pooled data from 8 trials demonstrate a small treatment benefit, interestingly detected as larger for radiographically diagnosed rhinosinusitis.[29] The benefit towards treatment likely represents selection bias toward sicker patients and should not encourage unnecessary use of imaging. Bacterial sinusitis is more likely if symptoms are severe, persistent, or worsen after an initial period of recovery (double sickening), and the CDC has advised that antibiotics be reserved for these situations. They recommend antibiotics be considered for patients with symptoms greater than 10 days, fever greater than 39°C, purulent nasal discharge or facial pain lasting more than 3 days, or with double sickening, that is, a worsening of symptoms after an initial improvement following a typical (5 day) viral illness.[7] If antibiotics are prescribed, coverage for ampicillin-resistant *H influenzae* and *Moraxella catarrhalis* (for example, with amoxicillin-clavulanate) should be considered.

Ultimately, the risks and benefits of antibiotics must be carefully weighed especially when the bias is to overuse. The CDC estimates that 47 million antibiotic courses or 30% of all antibiotics prescribed each year is for infections that do not require antibiotics.[30] Often, overly broad-spectrum antibiotics are given, and for longer than necessary courses.[31,32]

Inappropriate antibiotic usage is not benign. Approximately 145,000 annual visits to the emergency department are for adverse events from antibiotics. The majority (74%) of these reactions are allergic, with 24% reporting gastrointestinal (GI) disturbance and 9% requiring hospitalization.[33] *Clostridium* (or *Clostridioides*) *difficile* infection, which is highly associated with antibiotic usage, causes nearly 224,000 infections and 13,000 deaths annually. Finally, antibiotic overuse contributes to the growing problem of antibiotic resistance, with more than 2.8 million antibiotic-resistant infections and more than 35,000 deaths annually attributable to antibiotic resistant organisms.[34]

One reason clinicians might feel pressure to prescribe antibiotics despite the lack of supporting evidence is the sense that they have little else in terms of pharmacologic therapies to offer. Conservative management or symptomatic relief as a treatment plan often feels inadequate. However, navigating the many over-the-counter options is overwhelming, and patients need specific assistance and counseling. Formulations often include combinations of analgesics, antihistamines, decongestants, expectorants, and cough suppressants, and the average consumer needs medical advice on how to tailor their regimen.

ANALGESICS AND ANTIPYRETICS

Analgesics are commonly recommended for the headache, myalgias, and malaise associated with most URTIs. Historically, nonsteroidal anti-inflammatory drugs are touted to have better efficacy than acetaminophen. However, a pragmatic trial of close to 900 patients randomized to clinician advice on as-needed or around-the-clock paracetamol, ibuprofen, or both, found no inferiority in symptom relief between agents or type of usage.[35] The authors' experience supports the equivalency of both analgesics, and choice of one over the other is usually determined by the need to avoid specific toxicities (GI, renal, or hepatic).

ANTIHISTAMINES AND DECONGESTANTS

Rhinorrhea and congestion are sine qua non in URTIs, and antihistamine and decongestants are the mainstay of symptomatic therapies. Antihistamines address the swelling associated with increased vascular permeability; they reduce watery eyes, runny nose, itching, and sneezing. Decongestants mediate vasoconstriction of the upper respiratory vasculature, relieving nasal obstruction. Using the household sink as an analogy, antihistamines dial down the water flow, and decongestants unclog the drain.

In a systematic review, antihistamines performed best when taken early in the course of illness (first 2–4 days). Sedating antihistamines (diphenhydramine, chlorpheniramine) relieved symptoms better than nonsedating antihistamines (loratadine, cetirizine).[36]

Although decongestants (pseudoephedrine more than phenylephrine) reduce airway resistance and nasal congestion, they appear to be more powerful when combined with antihistamines.[37] A review of 27 trials totaling more than 5000 participants found more consistent symptom relief with this combination.[38] As a vasoconstrictor, decongestants can worsen hypertension and tachycardia, but this is less of a concern for the short courses necessary for treatment of acute URTIs; chronic use in perennial allergic rhinitis is more of a concern. Additional potential adverse effects of decongestants include tremors and other mild stimulatory effects, but only on a scale comparable to placebo.[37] Topical decongestants, such as oxymetazoline, should be limited to 2 to 3 days of use because rebound rhinitis can occur, making it very difficult for patients to wean themselves off this medication. Finally, there is some evidence to support the use of intranasal ipratropium[39] and intranasal steroids[40] for rhinorrhea and congestion, but these therapies require use for 2 weeks or more to be effective. Personally, the authors find that a good steaming, usually achieved in a hot shower by breathing in the mist for at least 10 minutes, achieves a decongesting benefit on par with a short-acting dose of a pharmacologic decongestant.

EXPECTORANTS AND COUGH SUPPRESSANTS

Persistent cough is one of the most troublesome and longest-lasting symptoms of URTIs. It is not common knowledge that the 2 mainstay therapies, expectorants and suppressants, approach cough management in conflicting ways. The former enhances the effectiveness of the cough, increasing mucous hydration and decreasing mucous viscosity to produce "juicier" coughs. In so doing, expectorants boost the respiratory system's reflex to rid itself of irritating sputum and debris. Guaifenesin, the only marketed expectorant in the United States, shortens the total duration of cough, but increases cough productivity and frequency.[41]

Cough suppressants do the exact opposite through peripheral and central inhibition of cough. Benzonatate, a peripheral agent, acts by anesthetizing stretch receptors in the lungs.[42] Dextromethorphan, as the D-isomer of the synthetic codeine analogue levorphanol, acts on the cough center in the brain's medulla. Both are effective in reducing cough intensity and frequency.[43] Central-acting cough suppressants can become drugs of abuse. Although this is commonly known for codeine and other traditional opioids, even dextromethorphan in high dosages can be misused for its euphoric and hallucinatory properties, often by younger individuals.

The authors' approach with patients is to explain the mechanisms of action for these 2 drug classes. If patients request assistance with bringing up phlegm and do not mind more intense coughing for a shorter duration of time, then guaifenesin is the natural choice. Most liquid formulations at 100 mg per teaspoon need to be dosed up to 600 mg/d or greater to achieve effect. If the patient's goal is to achieve relief from their cough during critical portions of their workday or at night to achieve uninterrupted sleep, the authors advise a cough suppressant.

NATURAL SUPPLEMENTS

Many patients turn to vitamins, herbs, and other dietary supplements to treat URTI symptoms. There is no evidence to support the use of the herb echinacea, garlic, or high doses of vitamin D for this purpose.[44] However, some limited evidence exists for the use of zinc, an essential mineral, postulated to inhibit rhinovirus replication. More than a dozen trials of various formulations of zinc (gluconate, acetate, sulfate) report shortened duration and reduced severity of cold symptoms. However, effective dosing requires administration every 2 hours and is limited by nausea.[45] In 2009, the Food and Drug Administration issued a warning against the use of intranasal zinc because of reported anosmia and a sensation of burning.[46] Vitamin C, an antioxidant, has long been considered to support the immune system and stave off colds. Dozens of clinical trials, however, fail to support this with the exception of a narrow subset of athletes (marathon runners, skiers, soldiers) for whom daily ingestion did demonstrate an up to 50% reduction in the frequency of colds. To reduce cold symptoms, at least 2 g of vitamin C daily is needed to achieve about an 8% benefit in adults.[47]

SUMMARY

In conclusion, URTIs are one of the most common challenges in ambulatory medicine. The number of symptoms associated with URTIs can feel bewildering, but focusing on the dominant set of symptoms and excluding the more morbid conditions is the authors' recommended approach. The key to achieving satisfactory outcomes for patients is proceeding in a systematic manner aimed at arriving at an accurate diagnosis. Thoughtful treatment requires an understanding of the limited utility of antibiotics and a generous allotment of time to advise patients on the numerous pharmacologic options for symptom management. Providing additional resources, such as a "viral prescription," that outlines possible diagnoses, general care instructions, and specific medication recommendations can empower patients to effectively self-manage. Viral prescriptions are available at the CDC or local Department of Health Web site in many languages.[48] These tools, along with close monitoring and ongoing communication, will help patients successfully navigate the course of their URTI.

CLINICS CARE POINTS

- A targeted history will reveal a dominant set of symptoms that often leads to accurate diagnosis.
- Clinical decision rules, such as the modified Centor criteria, can assist with accurate diagnosis of Group A Streptococcus pharyngitis.
- Antibiotics are not advised for acute uncomplicated bronchitis.
- There is a greater role for antibiotic therapy for adults with otitis media than for children.
- The majority of acute rhinosinusitis is viral in etiology however patients with more severe symptoms or with "double sickening" should be considered for antibacterials.
- There are many available treatments that target the symptoms of URTI, eg. cough, congestion, myalgias, and patients appreciate specific advice on how to navigate the multitude of options.
- For each specific type of upper respiratory infection there are several "don't miss" diagnoses that should always be on the provider's differential diagnosis list and should be effectively ruled out.

DISCLOSURE

The authors have nothing to disclose.

REFERENCES

1. National Ambulatory Medical Care Survey. National summary tables. 2016. Available at: https://www.cdc.gov/nchs/data/ahcd/namcs_summary/2016_namcs_web_tables.pdf. Accessed April 14, 2020.
2. Dixon RE. Economic costs of respiratory tract infections in the United States. Am J Med 1985;78(6B):45–51.
3. Harlan WR, Murt HA, Thomas JW, et al. Incidence, utilization, and costs associated with acute respiratory conditions, United States, 1980. Natl Med Care Util Expend Surv C 1986;(4):1–63.
4. Jiang F, Deng L, Zhang L, et al. Review of the clinical characteristics of coronavirus disease 2019 (COVID-19). J Gen Intern Med 2020. https://doi.org/10.1007/s11606-020-05762-w. Available at: https://doi.org/10.1007/s11606-020-05762-w. Accessed April 26, 2020.
5. Harmes KM, Blackwood RA, Burrows HL, et al. Otitis media: diagnosis and treatment. Am Fam Physician 2013;88(7):435–40.
6. Spurling GKP, Del Mar CB, Dooley L, et al. Delayed antibiotic prescriptions for respiratory infections. Cochrane Database Syst Rev 2017;(9):CD004417.
7. Harris AM, Hicks LA, Qaseem A. High Value Care Task Force of the American College of Physicians and for the Centers for Disease Control and Prevention. Appropriate antibiotic use for acute respiratory tract infection in adults: advice for high-value care from the American College of Physicians and the Centers for Disease Control and Prevention. Ann Intern Med 2016;164(6):425–34.
8. Rosenfeld RM, Piccirillo JF, Chandrasekhar SS, et al. Clinical practice guideline (update): adult sinusitis. Otolaryngol Head Neck Surg 2015;152(2 Suppl):S1–39.
9. Centor RM, Witherspoon JM, Dalton HP, et al. The diagnosis of strep throat in adults in the emergency room. Med Decis Making 1981;1:239–46.
10. McIsaac WJ, White D, Tannenbaum D, et al. A clinical score to reduce unnecessary antibiotic use in patients with sore throat. CMAJ 1998;158(1):75–83.
11. McIsaac WJ, Kellner JD, Aufricht P, et al. Empirical validation of guidelines for the management of pharyngitis in children and adults. JAMA 2004;291:1587–95.
12. Ebell MH, Smith MA, Barry HC, et al. Does this patient have strep throat? JAMA 2000;284(22):2912–8.
13. Pelucchi C, Grigoryan L, Galeone C, et al. Guideline for the management of acute sore throat. The ESCMID Sore Throat Guideline Group. Clin Microbiol Infect 2012; 18(Suppl 1):1.
14. Gottlieb M, Long B, Koyfman A. Clinical mimics: an emergency medicine-focused review of streptococcal pharyngitis mimics. J Emerg Med 2018;54: 619–29.
15. Alcaide ML, Bisno AL. Pharyngitis and epiglottitis. Infect Dis Clin North Am 2007; 21:449–69.
16. Glynn F, Fenton JE. Diagnosis and management of supraglottitis (epiglottitis). Curr Infect Dis Rep 2008;10(3):200–4.
17. Irwin RS, French CL, Chang AB, et al, CHEST Expert Cough Panel. Classification of cough as a symptom in adults and management algorithms: CHEST guideline and expert panel report. Chest 2018;153(1):196–209.
18. Albert RH. Diagnosis and treatment of acute bronchitis. Am Fam Physician 2010; 82(11):1345–50.
19. Altiner A, Wilm S, Däubener W, et al. Sputum colour for diagnosis of a bacterial infection in patients with acute cough. Scand J Prim Health Care 2009; 27(2):70–3.

20. Rapid diagnostic testing for influenza: information for clinical laboratory directors. Available at: https://www.cdc.gov/flu/professionals/diagnosis/rapidlab.htm. Accessed April 26, 2020.

21. Schuetz P, Wirz Y, Sager R, et al. Effect of procalcitonin-guided antibiotic treatment on mortality in acute respiratory infections: a patient level meta-analysis. Lancet Infect Dis 2018;18(1):95–107.

22. Metlay JP, Waterer GW, Long AC, et al. Diagnosis and treatment of adults with community-acquired pneumonia. An official clinical practice guideline of the American Thoracic Society and Infectious Diseases Society of America. Am J Respir Crit Care Med 2019;200(7):e45–67.

23. Cornia PB, Hersh AL, Lipsky BA, et al. Does this coughing adolescent or adult patient have pertussis? JAMA 2010;304(8):890–6.

24. Kenealy T, Arroll B. Antibiotics for the common cold and acute purulent rhinitis. Cochrane Database Syst Rev 2013;(6):CD000247.

25. Barnett M, Linder J. Antibiotic prescribing for adults with acute bronchitis in the United States 1996-2010. JAMA 2014;311(19):2020–2.

26. Smith S, Fahey T, Smucny J, et al. Antibiotics for acute bronchitis. Cochrane Database Syst Rev 2017;(6:):CD000245.

27. Schulman S, Bisno A, Clegg H, et al. Clinical practice guideline for the diagnosis and management of group A streptococcal pharyngitis: 2012 update by the Infectious Diseases Society of America. Clin Infect Dis 2012;55(10):1279–82.

28. Fairlie T, Shapiro D, Hersh A, et al. National trends in visit rates and antibiotic prescribing for adults with acute sinusitis. Arch Intern Med 2012;172(19):1513.

29. Lemiengre M, van Driel M, Merenstein D, et al. Antibiotics for acute rhinosinusitis in adults. Cochrane Database Syst Rev 2018;(9):CD006089.

30. CDC. Antibiotic use in the United States, 2018 update: progress and opportunities. Atlanta (GA): US Department of Health and Human Services, CDC; 2019.

31. Kabbani S, Hersh A, Shapiro D, et al. Opportunities to improve fluoroquinolone prescribing in the United States for adult ambulatory care visits. Clin Infect Dis 2018;67(1):134–6.

32. Kang L, Sanchez G, Bartoces M, et al. Antibiotic therapy duration in US adults with sinusitis. JAMA Intern Med 2018;178(7):992–4.

33. Geller A, Lovegrove M, Shehab N, et al. National estimates of emergency department visits for antibiotic adverse events among adults in the US, 2011-2015. J Gen Intern Med 2018;33(7):1060–8.

34. CDC. Antibiotic resistance threats in the United States, 2019. Atlanta (GA): U.S. Department of Health and Human Services, CDC; 2019.

35. Little P, Moore M, Kelly J, et al. Ibuprofen, paracetamol, and steam for patients with respiratory tract infections in primary care: pragmatic randomized factorial trial. BMJ 2013;347:6041–54.

36. De Sutter A, Saraswat A, van Driel M. Antihistamines for the common cold. Cochrane Database Syst Rev 2015;(11):CD009345.

37. Deckx L, De Sutter A, Guo L, et al. Nasal decongestants in monotherapy for the common cold. Cochrane Database Syst Rev 2016;(10):CD009612.

38. De Sutter A, van Driel M, Kumar A, et al. Oral anti-histamine-decongestant-analgesic combinations for the common cold. Cochrane Database Syst Rev 2012;(2):CD004976.

39. AlBalawi Z, Othman S, Alfakeh K. Intranasal ipratropium bromide for the common cold. Cochrane Database Syst Rev 2013;(6):CD008231.

40. Zalamanovici A, Yaphe J. Intranasal steroids for acute sinusitis. Cochrane Database Syst Rev 2013;(12):CD005149.

41. Albrecht H, Dicpinigaitis P, Guenin E. Role of guaifenesin in the management of chronic bronchitis and upper respiratory tract infections. Multidiscip Respir Med 2017;12:31–42.

42. Dicpinigastis P, Gayle Y, Solomon G, et al. Inhibition of cough-reflex sensitivity by benzonatate and guaifenesin in acute viral cough. Respir Med 2009;103(6): 902–6.

43. Yancy W, McCrory D, Coeytaux R, et al. Efficacy and tolerability of treatments for chronic cough: a systematic review and meta-analysis. Chest 2013;144(6): 1827–38.

44. Allan G, Arroll B. Prevention and treatment of the common cold: making sense of the evidence. CMAJ 2014;186(3):190–9.

45. Science M, Johnstone J, Roth D, et al. Zinc for the treatment of the common cold: a systematic review and meta-analysis of randomized controlled trials. CMAJ 2012;184(10):E551–61.

46. Harris G. FDA warns against use of popular cold remedy. New York, NY: New York Times; 2009. Available at: https://www.nytimes.com/2009/06/17/health/policy/ 17nasal.html. Accessed April 29, 2020.

47. Douglas R, Hemelia H, Chalker E, et al. Vitamin C for preventing and treating the common cold. Cochrane Database Syst Rev 2007;7.

48. New York State Department of Health. Viral prescription pad in multiple languages. 2018. Available at: https://www.health.ny.gov/professionals/protocols_ and_guidelines/antibiotic_resistance/viral_prescription_pad.htm. Accessed April 30, 2020.

Moving?

Make sure your subscription moves with you!

To notify us of your new address, find your **Clinics Account Number** (located on your mailing label above your name), and contact customer service at:

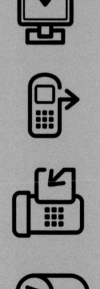

Email: journalscustomerservice-usa@elsevier.com

800-654-2452 (subscribers in the U.S. & Canada)
314-447-8871 (subscribers outside of the U.S. & Canada)

Fax number: 314-447-8029

Elsevier Health Sciences Division
Subscription Customer Service
3251 Riverport Lane
Maryland Heights, MO 63043

*To ensure uninterrupted delivery of your subscription, please notify us at least 4 weeks in advance of move.